Keto Copycat Recipies

Complete Step-by-Step Guide to Cooking Most Loved and Famous Restaurants Dishes and Losing Weight With the Ketogenic Diet

Victor Russo

made as to its accuracy or validity as the author has made no claims to be an expert on this topic. Notwithstanding, the reader is asked to do their own research and consult any subject matter experts they deem necessary to ensure the quality and accuracy of the material presented herein.

This statement is legally binding as deemed by the Committee of Publishers Association and the American Bar Association for the territory of the United States. Other jurisdictions may apply their own legal statutes. Any reproduction, transmission, or copying of this material contained in this work without the express written consent of the copyright holder shall be deemed as a copyright violation as per the current legislation in force on the date of publishing and the subsequent time thereafter. All additional works derived from this material may be claimed by the holder of this copyright.

The data, depictions, events, descriptions, and all other information forthwith are considered to be true, fair, and accurate unless the work is expressly described as a work of fiction. Regardless of the nature of this work, the Publisher is exempt from any responsibility of actions taken by the reader in conjunction with this work. The Publisher acknowledges that the reader acts of their own accord and releases the author and Publisher of any responsibility for the observance of tips, advice, counsel, strategies, and techniques that may be offered in this volume.

Table of Contents

INTRODUCTION

Congratulations on purchasing Keto Copycat Recipes, and thank you for doing so.

There are so many benefits of homemade food. Don't let anyone tell you homemade food is bland while you are on a ketogenic diet. This book will prove them wrong - with recipes from some of the most famous dishes, including restaurants and food establishments we all love. When you make these tasty dishes at home, you can make them suitable for your health needs.

You are opening a new world to keto-friendly recipes. If you are not aware of how the keto diet works, don't worry because you will be introduced to tons of factual information and recipes.

Following a nutritious diet, such as the keto plan, it is essential for your overall well-being. You can stick to the ingredients you want to include in your recipes. Moreover, cooking your favorite dishes at home gives you total control over what you are eating. You can maintain not only a healthy body but also a satisfied mind. Cooking your meals at home will also ensure that you can keep your calorie consumption in check.

I hope you find all the information you need to drop those unwanted pounds while enjoying your favorite meals and treats! Have some fun with your newly found ways of dining. Let's now see how it all works!

CHAPTER 1: THE KETO DIET COMPOSITION

The ketogenic diet brings you many benefits with its low-carbohydrates and high-fat content. It shares many similarities with the Atkins diet with its low-carb factors. However, it is simpler than Adkins, since you have to follow four phases with Adkins. With keto, you begin 'winning' on day one.

A ketogenic diet necessitates drastically decreasing the intake of carbohydrates and switching it with fat. Due to this reduction in carbohydrates, your body enters a metabolic state known as ketosis. When ketosis takes place, your body starts burning fat for energy efficiency, which converts the fats into ketones in your liver. This transition provides energy and more power to the brain.

The "ketogenic" or "keto" diet is so named because it results in the production of small fuel molecules by your body, which is called "ketones." These ketones act as an alternate fuel source in your body, which can be used when glucose (blood sugar) is in short supply.

Ketones are produced from fats by your liver when you consume very few calories or very few carbs. These ketones then act as a source of fuel for your brain and the rest of your body. The brain requires a lot of energy to function every day. It can directly run only on ketones or glucose but not on fats.

When you start a keto diet, your entire body turns to fat as the fuel source and burns fat twenty-four-seven. When the insulin levels in your body get extremely low, the burning of fat can increase significantly. It becomes possible for your body to gain access to the stored fats to burn them off.

Ketogenic Diet Varieties

Available variations of the ketogenic technique include:

- **Targeted Keto Diet (TKD)** – This version of the ketogenic diet lets you include carbs when you work out.

- **Cyclical Keto Diet (CKD)** – This version includes allotments of higher-carbohydrate refeeds, like two high-carb days following five ketogenic days.

- **Standard Keto Diet (SDK)** – This is a high-fat, medium protein allotments, and very low-carb diet. It generally contains only five percent carbs, twenty percent protein, and seventy-five percent fats.

- **High-Protein Keto Diet** – This diet has similarities with a standard keto diet; however, it includes more protein. It generally contains five percent carbs, thirty-five percent protein, and sixty percent fats.

The Science Behind Keto Diets

A keto diet allows your body to reach a status called ketosis. It is a metabolic shift in which your body burns fats instead of carbs as its primary fuel source. Even though the definition seems pretty simple, it is essential to know how the body uses energy to understand how the keto diet works and its benefits.

Generally, when you consume carbs in your diet, they get converted into insulin and glucose.

- Glucose is the preferred energy source of your body. This is because it is the simplest form of sugar and can be easily converted by your body to be used as energy.

- Insulin is a hormone that is secreted by the pancreas. It processes the glucose present in your blood and transports it throughout the body to where it is required. Insulin converts glucose to fat (adipose tissue) for later use when the energy levels are sufficient.

In typical high-carbohydrate diets, the primary energy source is glucose because there is an abundance of it. But, only a limited amount of glucose can be stored by the body. It is only enough to last for a few days. Thus, if you stop eating carbs for a couple of days, your body undergoes a biochemical process called ketogenesis and starts relying on other forms of energy.

The liver will begin to break down fats as a usable energy source through the ketogenesis process - rather than carbohydrates. The ketone bodies or ketones are produced as an alternate source of energy to glucose. When ketogenesis starts, the levels of ketones are increased, and the body is in ketosis.

Foods to Eat on a Keto Diet

When you're on a keto diet, you should base most of your meals around these foods:

- **Seafood** – Seafood like fish and shellfish are incredibly ketofriendly. Fatty fish include mackerel, tuna, trout, and salmon; all are high in selenium, potassium, and B vitamins, yet virtually free of carbohydrates. These fatty fish are rich in omega-three fatty acids. They have been found to reduce insulin levels and increase insulin sensitivity in obese and overweight individuals. However, the amount of carbohydrates varies in different types of shellfish. For example, even though shrimp and most crabs don't contain carbohydrates, other shellfish varieties do. While you can still include shellfish in your diet, be sure to account for those carbohydrates if you're trying to maintain a limit. Try to eat at least two servings of seafood every week.

- **Cheese** – Cheese is delicious as well as nutritious. There are more than a hundred different varieties of cheese. Many of them are rich in fats and low in carbohydrates, making them an excellent choice for the ketogenic diet. Unprocessed cheese has a high content of saturated fats and conjugated linoleic acid. It has been linked to improvement in body composition and weight loss and protection against heart diseases.

- **Avocados** – Choose an avocado since they are incredibly healthy and are rich in several minerals and vitamins. Moreover, as they are rich in potassium, consuming avocados can help transition to a more manageable ketogenic diet. One-half or 3.5 ounces of a medium-sized avocado contains only about two grams of carbohydrates. Studies reveal that avocados can also help improve the levels of triglyceride and cholesterol.

- **Meat & Poultry** – The two options are considered a staple food for people on a keto diet. Fresh meat and poultry are good sources of Vitamin B, high-quality protein, and minerals such as zinc, selenium, and potassium and don't contain any carbohydrates. They can help to preserve muscle mass as you pass through the phases of the keto diet.

- **Eggs** – Eggs are an ideal food for a keto lifestyle, as one large egg has less than six grams of protein and less than one gram of carbohydrates. Eggs can also help maintain stable blood sugar levels and trigger hormones that can increase satiety feelings. Therefore, it can lead to lower calorie intake for about twentyfour hours. The majority of an egg's nutrients, including the antioxidants zeaxanthin and lutein, are present in the yolk. So, enjoy a whole egg as desired.

- **Low-Carb Vegetables** – Non-starchy vegetables are rich in nutrients, such as Vitamin C, but low in calories and carbohydrates. They contain fiber, which cannot be digested and absorbed by your body like other carbohydrates. A majority of vegetables are low in carbs. However, eating even one serving of vegetables like beets, yams, and potatoes that contain starch can put you over your carbohydrate limit for the day. For nonstarchy vegetables, one cup of raw spinach contains less than one gram of carbohydrates. Whereas, one cup of cooked Brussels sprouts has about eight grams of carbs. They also contain antioxidants that can protect against unstable free radicals that can damage your cells.

- **Nuts & Seeds** – They are incredibly healthy and high in fats and low in carbohydrates. Studies have shown that consuming nuts frequently can decrease the risk of depression, certain types of cancers, heart diseases, and other chronic diseases. Moreover, seeds and nuts are rich sources of fiber, which can absorb fewer calories overall and also help you feel full.

Benefits of Keto Diets

You can consider ketogenic diets as a super-charged, low-carb diet that maximizes the health benefits. Several studies reveal the reasons behind why a keto diet is better than a low-fat diet.

Some of the reasons include increased consumption of proteins, which has several health benefits. The improved insulin sensitivity reduced blood sugar levels, and increased ketones might also play a key role.

Assist With Weight Loss

Following a keto diet is an effective way to reduce the risk factors for diseases and lose weight. One research revealed that people who used the keto diet lost about two times more weight versus those who followed a low-fat and calorie-restricted diet.

Appetite Control

You are more likely to have better control over your appetite when following a keto diet. Studies have proved that it is prevalent for hunger feelings to reduce drastically when on a keto plan. This trend tends to make it easier to eat less and lose extra weight. It also makes it easier to follow intermittent fasting. In turn, it can increase your efforts to speed up your weight loss and reverse type 2 diabetes, beyond the effects of just keto.

Not having to fight the feelings of hunger can also help with food or sugar addiction. Lastly, satiety can be part of the solution. Food can become whatever you prefer – your friend, or just fuel.

Reversal of Type 2 Diabetes & Control of Blood Sugar

Impaired insulin factor, high blood sugar, and changes in metabolism are characteristics of diabetes. Following a keto diet can help you lose extra weight - directly linked with metabolic syndrome, pre-diabetes, and type 2 diabetes.

One research showed that the keto diet could improve the sensitivity to insulin by almost seventy-five percent. Another study conducted on individuals with type 2 diabetes showed that seven out of the twenty-one participants could discontinue all diabetes medicines.

In another study, a group of people who followed the keto diet lost about twenty-four pounds - while people who followed a high-carb diet lost only fifteen pounds. This is an essential benefit when considering the connection between type 2 diabetes and weight. In the keto group, 95.2 percent of people were able to discontinue or decrease diabetes medication usage - compared to only sixty-two percent in the high-carb group.

Improved Health Markers

Several studies reveal that keto diets can improve many important risk factors for heart diseases, such as cholesterol profiles. The cholesterol profile includes triglycerides and HDL or high-density lipoprotein cholesterol. The levels of LDL or low-density lipoprotein cholesterol are also moderately impacted. It also generally improves blood pressure, insulin level, and blood sugar levels.

Such commonly improved health markers are linked to metabolic syndrome. The keto diet can effectively treat this insulin-resistant condition.

Energy & Mental Performance

Keto diets can improve your energy and mental performance. Your brain doesn't require dietary carbs when you're on a keto diet. It is fueled by ketones twenty-four-seven, as well as a minimal amount of glucose produced by your liver. It doesn't need any dietary carbohydrates.

As a result, ketosis causes a steady flow of ketones to the brain as fuel. This helps avoid any problems related to big blood sugar swings. This also could result in improved mental clarity, brain fog resolution, and improved concentration and focus.

More Possible Keto Benefits

The Keto diet was initially used for the treatment of neurological problems like epilepsy. Research studies have also revealed that the keto diet can help improve several health conditions, such as:

- Brain injuries

- Heart diseases

- Epilepsy

- Cancer

- Parkinson's disease

- Alzheimer's disease

- Polycystic ovary syndrome

- Acne

The keto diet can work 'only if' you're consistent and stick with the diet for a long time. It is especially beneficial for diabetic or obese individuals or those wanting to improve his/her metabolic health.

CHAPTER 2: COPYCAT RECIPES - KETO BREAKFAST

Bacon Temptation Omelet From IHOP

Total Prep & Cooking Time: 13 minutes

Yields: One Serving

Nutrition Facts: Calories: 1473 | Protein: 69g | Carbs: 27g | Fat: 119g | Fiber: 0.01g

Ingredients:

- 4 eggs

- 6 slices - divided

- ¼ cup of shredded Monterey Jack Cheese

- 4 oz. of American cheese

- 2 tbsp. milk - divided for use

- Optional: 2 tbsp. of pancake batter (prepare a small amount of pancake batter if you desire)

Method:

1. Preheat a skillet or griddle to 350 degrees Fahrenheit.

2. Cook the bacon and set it aside. When it's cooled a bit, break it apart.

3. Arrange the American cheese in a saucepan.

4. Add one tablespoon of milk into the pan and heat the saucepan over a medium flame.

5. Stir the cheese and milk continuously with a wooden spoon until the cheese melts to form a smooth cheese sauce.

6. Adjust the flame to a low level and stir until the cheese sauce thickens.

7. Break the eggs into a mixing container. Add bacon bits from four slices of cooked bacon, the remaining tablespoon of milk, and pancake batter. Vigorously whisk until everything blends smoothly.

8. Lightly spritz a skillet or griddle or skillet using a bit of cooking oil spray. Pour the mixture of eggs, bacon, pancake batter, and milk into the griddle in a rectangular shape. As the mixture is cooked, the omelet is formed.

9. When the omelet is almost prepared, pour half of the cheese sauce over the omelet and roll it. Sprinkle cheese and remaining small pieces of bacon on the top of the omelet.

10. Your bacon temptation omelet from IHOP is ready to serve. Serve it with the remaining cheese sauce on its side if desired.

Cheese Toast at Sizzler Restaurant

Total Prep & Cooking Time: 15 minutes

Yields: 12 Servings

Nutrition Facts: Calories: 255 | Protein: 7g | Carbs: 12g | Fat: 19g

Ingredients:

- 12 slices pre-sliced soft white bread

- 1 cup unchilled butter

- 1 ½ cups grated parmesan cheese

Method:

1. Whip the butter using a stand mixer or by hand until it's fluffy.

2. Fold in the cheese and whip until combined (1-2 min.).

3. Spread a thick layer of the mixture over each bread slice.

4. Warm a large skillet using the medium-high-temperature setting.

5. Arrange the slices buttered side down and heat for one to two minutes until the butter and cheese spread is golden, and the backside is softened.

Notes: Add a portion of garlic (1 minced clove) mixed into the cheese butter for a garlic hit. Dried herbs are a plus, including parsley, oregano, or rosemary.

Cranberry Bliss Bars

Total Prep & Cooking Time: 35 minutes

Yields: 16 Servings

Nutrition Facts: Calories: 110 | Protein: 2g | Carbs: 3g | Fat: 10g | Fiber: 1g

Ingredients:

- ⅓ cup your favorite sweetener

- 6 tbsp. unchilled-softened butter

- 1 pinch salt

- 1 tsp. molasses

- 2 eggs

- ½ tsp. orange extract

- 1 tsp. vanilla

- ¼ cup each coconut & almond flour

- 1 tsp. of baking powder

- ¼ cup ground golden flax (or more almond flour)

- Optional: ¼ tsp. ginger

- 1 cup fresh cranberries + ½ tsp. pure stevia

The Frosting:

- 4 drops - lemon extract

- 4 oz. unchilled cream cheese

- 1 tbsp. unchilled butter

- ½ cup powdered sweetener

- Also Needed: 8x8 baking pan/dish

Method:

1. Warm the oven to reach 350 degrees Fahrenheit. Grease the baking tray/dish.

2. Cream the butter and sweetener. Mix in the molasses with the eggs, salt, and extracts until thoroughly incorporated.

3. Mix in the dry fixings and thoroughly combine.

4. Finely chop the cranberries by hand or in a food processor. Toss it with ½ teaspoon of Stevia. Fold in the cranberries.

5. Spread the mixture into the baking dish. Bake it until it's golden brown (30-35 min.). Let it cool for 15 minutes.

6. Meanwhile, combine the cream cheese with the butter, sweetener, and lemon extract until fluffy.

7. Gently spread the icing over the cooled bars.

8. Slightly cool the bars and drop small portions of icing over the tops. Top it off using chopped fresh cranberries mixed with sweetener.

9. Pop the container into the fridge until cold and cut into squares to serve.

Egg and Cheese Protein Box From Starbucks

Total Prep & Cooking Time: 5 minutes

Yields: One Serving

Nutrition Facts: Calories: 602| Protein: 34g | Carbs: 16g | Fat: 17g | Fiber: 3g

Ingredients:

- 2 oz. of grapes

- 2 hard-boiled eggs

- 1 tbsp. peanut butter

- ½ apple - sliced

- 2 oz. white cheddar cheese

- 1 slice multigrain muesli bread

Method:

1. In the meal prep container of your choice, add and combine all the ingredients.

2. Serve.

Keto Donuts From Krispy Kreme

Total Prep & Cooking Time: 30 minutes

Yields: Six Servings

Nutrition Facts: Calories: 168 | Protein: 4.8g | Carbs: 5.5g | Fat: 11.3g | Fiber: 4.5g

Ingredients:

Donut Ingredients:

- ½ cup almond flour

- ¼ cup keto-friendly protein powder

- 2 tbsp. coconut flour

- ¼ cup Swerve

- ⅛ to ¼ cup of unsweetened vanilla almond milk

- 2 eggs

- ¼ tsp. salt

- 2 tsp. baking powder

- 1 tsp. of vanilla

Glaze Ingredients:

- ¼ cup Swerve

- ¼ cup grass-fed butter

- 1 tsp. vanilla

Method:

Donuts Instructions:

1. Warm the oven at 350 degrees Fahrenheit.

2. Whisk to mix each of the six donut ingredients in a large bowl until smooth.

3. Spray coconut oil spray on the donut pan. Spoon the dough into a frosting bag or a quart-sized bag to pipe out the dough into the donut pan filling two-thirds of it.

4. Set a timer to bake the donuts for 14-16 minutes or until the donuts get lightly browned.

Glaze Instructions:

1. Let the donuts cool completely.

2. Melt the glaze ingredients over medium heat until it's well mixed.

3. Remove the glaze from the heat.

4. Cool and dip the donuts into the glaze to serve.

Eggs Benedict at Delmonico's Restaurant

Total Prep & Cooking Time: 5 minutes

Yields: Four Servings

Nutrition Facts: Calories: 190 | Protein: 5g | Carbs: 1g | Fat: 18g | Fiber: 0g

Ingredients:

Low-Carb Muffins (per person)

- 2 egg whites

- 1 tbsp. melted butter

- 1 tbsp. almond meal/flour

- ¼ tsp. baking powder **Poached Eggs:**

- 1 cup water

- 1 egg (per person)

- *Hollandaise Sauce (per person)*

- ½ tbsp. lemon juice

- 2 egg yolks

- 4 tbsp. unsalted butter

- Optional: ¼ tsp. salt - do not use if using salted butter

Extra Ingredients (each person)

- 1-2 slices - Canadian bacon/ham

- Optional: 2-4 spinach leaves

Also Needed:

- Instant Pot & Accessories Pack

- Ramekins or coffee mugs

Method:

The Muffins:

1. Measure and add the butter into a ramekin to melt. Pop it into the microwave briefly (10 to 15 seconds.

2. Whisk in the baking powder and almond flour.

3. Break the eggs and separate the yolk from the white. Toss the whites into the batter. Save the egg yolks for the hollandaise sauce.

4. Thoroughly incorporate the muffin batter and pop it into the microwave for 1 ½ minutes. The muffin will rise as it cooks but will recede as it cools.

5. After the muffin is cooled, gently loosen the edges using a butter knife. Remove it from the ramekin.

6. Cool the muffin and slice it in half to toast.

Poach the Eggs:

7. Pour one cup of water into the Instant Pot, arranging the trivet in the bottom.

8. Lightly grease the muffin liners, silicone trays, or ramekins. Crack an egg into each cup. Cover the container with foil and lower it onto the trivet in the Instant Pot.

9. Securely close the lid and seal the pressure valve. Set the timer for one to two minutes using the manual - pressure cook setting. Once the time is up, quick- release the pressure and remove the eggs.

Prepare the Sauce:

10. Blend the egg yolks with the lemon juice and salt in a blender.

11. While the blender is running, slowly add the hot melted butter into the blender from the top. Mix it for about ½ of a minute and turn it off.

To Assemble:

12. Make your plate. Toast the muffin and place the half on the plate.

13. Layer the spinach, meat of choice, and the egg on top. Drizzle a spoonful of the freshly prepared sauce over the top and serve.

Notes: **You will also use one cup of water in the cooker - no matter how many eggs you are preparing. Keep in mind, each ingredient for the dish is shown per person.

Poach as many eggs and fixings as desired.

Keto Everything Bagel From Starbucks

Total Prep & Cooking Time: 29 minutes

Yields: Six Bagels

Nutrition Facts: Calories: 449 | Protein: 27.8g | Carbs: 10g | Fat: 35.5g | Fiber: 4g

Ingredients:

- 2 cups - almond flour

- 3 cups - low-moisture shredded mozzarella cheese

- 3 large eggs - divided

- 5 tbsp. cream cheese

- 1 tsp. onion powder

- 1 tbsp. baking powder

- 3 tbsp. Everything Bagel Seasoning

- 1 tsp. garlic powder

- 1 tsp. dried Italian seasoning

- Also Needed: Rimmed baking sheet

Method:

1. Warm the oven at 425 degrees Fahrenheit.

2. Prepare the baking tray using a silicone baking mat. You can also use a parchment paper, alternatively.

3. Combine the almond flour, onion powder, garlic powder, baking powder, and dried Italian seasoning in a mixing container. Stir well until everything thoroughly combines.

4. Break one egg into a small bowl and beat it with a wooden spoon. The beaten egg will be used to brush the top of the bagels.

5. Mix the cream cheese and mozzarella cheese in a large bowl. Choose a bowl that can be used in the microwave oven. Microwave the mixture of cheeses for 1 ½ minutes. Remove the bowl to stir the water and egg yolk thoroughly. Blend till a small dough ball is formed.

6. Keep in the refrigerator for ½ hour.

7. Set the oven temperature at 375 degrees Fahrenheit to warm.

8. *Blind Bake the Crust – Large Pan Instructions*: Line the baking sheet with parchment paper. Make a circle with the dough by rolling. Roll loosely and don't leave cracks. Moving it around the rolling pin should be - hence - done with care. You do not want gaps in the crust.

9. On the dough, place a parchment paper, and bake this crust for 15-20 minutes.

10. Don't make it too brown, and let cool. Add the cheese, bacon, and ham slices.

11. *Quiche Filling- Large Pan Instructions:* Add two of each (egg yolks and whole eggs). Whisk them in a mixing container and mix in the milk and heavy cream.

12. When the crust turns cold, mix the custard mixture, and blend it well. Pour it into the shell. Cook in the oven for 50 minutes, after bringing down the temperature to 350 degrees Fahrenheit. When the quiche wiggles, transfer it to the countertop. When cooled, it gets set.

13. *Crust: Small Pan Instructions:* Make the crust in the food processor. First, add flour, then salt, followed by the butter—pulse for a few seconds. Pour water and add the yolk. Blend till you get a small ball dough.

14. The oven should be preheated to 375 degrees Fahrenheit. For the smaller sized crust, you need to prepare four to five rounds of the dough. Poke with a fork five times to prevent misshaping while you bake the crust.

15. Bake the crust for ten minutes. The crust should not turn overly brown. Now, bring down the oven temperature to 350 degrees Fahrenheit. Wait till the shells are completely cooled. Now, add ham, cheese, and bacon in equal amounts.

16. *Quiche Filling: Small Pan Instructions:* In a bowl, place the two whole eggs. Then place the egg yolks. To it, add heavy cream

and milk. Stir this thoroughly, and all the ingredients should be blended completely.

17. Fill the quiche with the egg custard. Now, let it get baked for 35 minutes. Wait till the quiche to wiggle. When it wiggles slightly, take it off from the oven. Cool it. When it cools completely, it is set.

Sausage & Egg McMuffin Breakfast Sandwich

Total Prep & Cooking Time: 15 minutes

Yields: One Serving

Nutrition Facts: Calories: 880 | Protein: 32g | Carbs: 8g | Fat: 82g | Fiber: 2g

Ingredients:

- 2 large-sized eggs

- 1 tbsp. butter

- 1 tbsp. mayonnaise

- 2 cooked sausage patties (see recipe)

- 2 slices - cheese - sharp cheddar

- Avocado slices

Method:

1. Prepare a large skillet using the medium-temperature setting to melt the butter. Lightly oil silicone egg molds or mason jar rings and add them to the pan.

2. Break each of the eggs into the rings and use a fork to break the yolks gently.

3. Place a lid on the skillet and cook until the eggs are cooked as desired (3-4 min.). Transfer the eggs from the rings.

4. Place one of the eggs on a plate. Add half of the mayo. Top it with one of the sausage patties, a slice of cheese, and avocado.

5. Arrange the second sausage patty over the avocado and sprinkle on the rest of the cheese. Spread the rest of the mayo on the second cooked egg and top it off with cheese.

6. Serve and forget about the restaurant (for now).

Spinach & Cheese Egg Souffle From Panera

Total Prep & Cooking Time: 35 minutes

Yields: Four Servings

Nutrition Facts: Calories: 513 | Protein: 21g | Carbs: 24g | Fat: 37g | Fiber: 1g

Ingredients:

- 8 oz. can of Pillsbury rolls - butter flake crescent type

- 6 large eggs (1 for egg wash)

- 3 tbsp. finely chopped fresh spinach

- 2 tbsp. milk

- 2 tbsp. heavy cream

- ¼ cup - each kind of cheese:

- Asiago cheese

- Monterey Jack cheese

- Sharp Cheddar cheese

- 1 tbsp. Parmesan cheese

- 4 bacon slices

- ¼ tsp. salt

Method:

1. Warm the oven in advance to reach 375 degrees Fahrenheit.

2. Cook the bacon until it's crispy and break it into small bits.

3. In a medium-sized microwaveable bowl, break five eggs. Add the cheddar cheese, parmesan cheese, Monterey Jack cheese, heavy cream, milk, bacon, salt, and spinach into the bowl. Stir and thoroughly combine. Microwave the mixture for thirty seconds.

4. Take the bowl from the microwave, stir well, and put it back into the oven to microwave the mixture for 20 seconds. Repeat the process four to five times until the mixture is thickened. You will find the mixture is still runny and appears to be uncooked after several process repetitions. However, the combination process will help you hold up the crescent roll dough when you fold it over the top.

5. Unfold and separate the crescent roll dough into four rectangular pieces. Press the perforated line in between the triangles to form the rectangle. Roll out all four rectangles separately until they get a measurement of six square-inches each.

6. Spray four souffle dishes or ramekins about four-five inches in diameter with cooking spray. Place one rolled out crescent roll in each of the souffle dishes with edges of roll hanging over the sides.

7. Pour one-third cup of microwaved egg mixture on top of each rolled dough. Sprinkle a small amount of Asiago cheese, dividing one-fourth of the whole amount on top of each souffle dish's microwaved egg mixture. Fold four corners of the crescent roll over the top of the egg mixture.

8. Break the remaining egg into a mixing container and beat with a wooden spoon to make the egg wash. Brush the egg with a pastry brush over the top of each folded crescent roll dough.

9. Set a timer to bake the dough for twenty minutes at 375 degrees Fahrenheit until the top gets brown.

Strawberry Pancake Puppies From Denny's

Total Prep & Cooking Time: 20-25 minutes

Yields: Eight Servings

Nutrition Facts: Calories: 355| Protein: 3g | Carbs: 20g| Fat: 26g | Fiber: 1g

Ingredients:

For Pancake Puppies:

- 1 cup of water

- 2 cups of pancake mix – choose the type that requires only water to be added

- 3 tbsp. strawberry preserves

- Oil –to fry

- 2 tbsp. of white chocolate chips

For Cheesecake Dip:

- 2 oz. of cream cheese

- 2 oz. of butter

- ¼ tsp. vanilla

- ¾ cup of powdered sugar

Method:

- Heat the vegetable oil, keeping the temperature to 350 degrees Fahrenheit.

- In a fine wire sieve, add the berries and keep it under running water. Only the strawberries should be left. Then, mince the strawberries.

- Mix the pancake mix using minced strawberry preserves, white chocolate chips, and water. Blend them thoroughly by stirring.

- Drop the batter in portions into the oil. You can use a oneounce cookie scoop for this.

- The pancake puppies should become brown at the bottom. Flip them and cook for 30 minutes more.

- Take them from the oil and place them on a layer of paper towels to drain for a few minutes.

- Sprinkle the cake puppies using a dash of powdered sugar. Serve the puppies along with cream cheese frosting.

- *For Cheesecake Dip*: Mix cream cheese, vanilla, butter, and powdered sugar in a small-sized bowl. Use a mixer to blend them thoroughly until you make the frosting smooth.

Waffle House Keto Waffles

Total Prep & Cooking Time: 30 minutes

Yields: Five Servings

Nutrition Facts: Calories: 277.2 | Protein: 6.8 g | Carbs: 4.6 g | Fat: 25.6g | Fiber: 2.1 g

Ingredients:

- 5 eggs - medium

- 4 tbsp. coconut flour

- 4 tbsp./to taste - granulated sweetener of choice

- 1 tsp. baking powder

- 2 tsp. vanilla

- 3 tbsp. keto-friendly** milk or cream

- 1 stick + 1 tbsp./125g of butter - melted

Method:

1. Separate the eggs and whisk the egg whites to create stiff peaks.

2. In another container, combine the egg yolks with the sweetener, baking powder, and coconut flour.

3. Melt the butter and slowly mix it into the batter mixture. Pour and mix in the vanilla and milk.

4. Fold spoonfuls of the whisked egg whites into the yolk mixture.

5. Pour the waffle mixture into the heated waffle maker and cook until it's nicely browned. Continue the process until all of the batter has been prepared.

Note: ** The original recipe calls for full-fat milk, but it is best if you choose keto-friendly options, such as almond, soy, or coconut milk.

CHAPTER 3: COPYCAT KETO CHICKEN RECIPES FOR LUNCH

Broccoli Cheddar Chicken From Cracker Barrel

Total Prep & Cooking Time: 45 minutes

Yields: Four Servings

Nutrition Facts: Calories: 690 | Protein: 40g | Carbs: 20g | Fats: 44g | Fiber: 5g

Ingredients:

½ tsp. salt

1 cup of milk

½ tsp. paprika

8 oz. frozen chopped broccoli

½ tsp. pepper

4 chicken breast – boneless and skinless

1 can of cheddar cheese soup

1 ½ cups of crushed Ritz crackers

6 oz. cheddar cheese- shredded

Method:

1. Start by preheating the oven. Set the oven temperature at 350 degrees Fahrenheit. Grease a casserole dish slightly.

2. Mix salt and pepper. Use it to season the chicken and keep the chicken aside in a prepared dish.

3. Use a medium-sized bowl, add the milk, paprika, soup, and cheddar cheese. Mix them thoroughly.

4. On the chicken, pour about half of the cream mixture and a dash of the broccoli pieces.

5. Use the Ritz cracker pieces and cheese mixture as the topping.

6. Bake it for 45 minutes in the preheated oven.

Note: For a crunchy topping, mixer the cracker crumbs with melted butter of one or two tbsp. Sprinkle this over the top.

Chicken Bake From Costco

Total Prep & Cooking Time: 40 minutes

Yields: Six Servings

Nutrition Facts: Calories: 571 | Protein: 30g | Carbs: 19g | Fats: 41g

Ingredients:

- ½ cup of parmesan

- 3 cups of mozzarella cheese

- 1 cup of bacon crisps

- 2 cups of cooked chicken

- 1 ½ lb. pizza dough

- Flour

- 1 cup of Ranch dressing

Method:

1. Divide the dough into six parts.

2. Roll them into rectangular shapes. Leaving about an inch on all the sides, apply the ranch on the rolled dough. Top the dough with bacon and chicken

3. Place a handful of mozzarella cheese. Roll the dough slowly. Use a baking sheet and grease it with oil. Place the rolls one by one carefully on the baking sheet greased with oil.

4. On the outside of the rolls, apply the ranch in a small quantity using a brush.

5. Set a timer to bake at 415 degrees Fahrenheit (17-20 min.). When the time is over, transfer the pan to the stovetop.

6. Sprinkle them using a portion of the parmesan cheese on the rolls. Again, bake the rolls in the oven. Do not bake for more than five minutes. Keep in mind that you need to get golden brown rolls.

7. Serve immediately - while the cheese is in a melted state.

Note: The pizza dough should be purchased or made before you start making the recipe. If you are using full-portion pizza dough, double the recipe, or save the rest of the dough in the refrigerator for another time.

Chicken Casserole From Cracker Barrel

Total Prep & Cooking Time: 50 minutes

Yields: Six Servings

Nutrition Facts: Calories: 457 | Protein: 45g | Carbs: 6g | Fat: 27g | Fiber: 2g

Ingredients:

The Cornbread:

- ⅓ cup of flour - all-purpose

- 1 ½ tsp. baking powder

- 1 cup yellow cornmeal

- ½ tsp. - salt

- 1 tbsp. sugar

- ¾ cup of buttermilk

- 1 egg

- ½ tsp. baking soda

- ½ cup of butter - melted

The Filling:

- 2 ½ cups of chicken breast

- ¼ cup of yellow onion

- ½ cup celery

- 1 ¾ cups of chicken broth

- 2 tbsp. butter o oz. can of cream of chicken soup

- 1 tsp. salt

- ¼ tsp. pepper

Method:

1. Do the Prep: Chop the chicken into bite-sized pieces. Thinly slice the celery and chop the onion.

2. For Cornbread: In a mixing bowl, whisk the yellow cornmeal, all-purpose flour, egg, buttermilk, baking soda, vegetable oil, sugar, salt, and baking powder. Combine thoroughly to form a smooth mixture.

3. Grease an eight-inch square baking pan. Pour the batter into it. At 375 degrees Fahrenheit, bake in the oven. The time should be around 20-25 minutes. Or - bake till the batter turns golden brown. When it is finished, transfer the bread to the countertop and let it cool.

4. When the cornbread is completely cool, you need to crumble all of it. Then - take three cups of the cornbread crumbles and toss them into a mixing container. Mix in the melted butter to the crumbles. Mix thoroughly and set it aside.

5. For Chicken Filling: You need a pan of medium size. Heat in the flame of medium to a high level. Add the butter into it, and heat it. Sauté the chopped celery and onions in this pan until they are translucent.

6. Now to the pan, add the cream of chicken soup, pepper, salt, and chicken broth. Keep stirring. The ingredients should be thoroughly blended. Stir till the soup is completely dissolved.

7. Add the cooked chicken into this pan. Continue stirring until everything blends using a low simmer. Keep cooking for another five minutes. After that, take the pan off from the stove.

8. Use a casserole dish or four individual casserole dishes. Butter the container/dishes, and place the chicken filling into them.

9. Generously scatter the cornbread crumbles over the chicken mixture. (Never stir the chicken filling. All you need to do is to form a crust on that filling.)

10. Preheat an oven at 350 degrees Fahrenheit. Set a timer and bake it for about thirty-five to f35-40 minutes. This ensures the crumbles turn golden yellow. Place the baking dish into the oven.

11. Remove when done. Serve when hot.

Note: Substitute cream of mushroom or potato soup instead of the cream of chicken soup if desired.

Chipotle Chicken

Total Prep & Cooking Time: 18 hours 15 minutes

Yields: Eight Servings

Nutrition Facts: Calories: 293 | Protein: 24.9g | Carbs: 5.8g | Fats: 18.7g | Fibre: 2.1 g

Ingredients:

☐ 1 oz. each:

o Dried ancho chili pepper o

Dried chipotle chili pepper

● 4 garlic cloves

43

- ½ red onion

- 2 tbsp. of olive oil

- ½ cup of water • 1 tsp. each:

  o Black pepper (freshly ground)

  o Dried oregano o Ground

  cumin

- lb. of chicken thighs (boneless & skinless)

- 2 tsp. of sea salt

Method:

1. Grab a bowl and in it, add the two types of chile peppers. Mix in the water. Allow the peppers to become softened for about 12 hours. After that, remove the peppers and eliminate the seeds.

2. Use the bowl of a blender and, in it, add red onion, chile peppers, cumin, sea salt, garlic, black pepper, and oregano. Blend everything until you get a coarse paste. Add the olive oil and blend again until it reaches a smooth mixture.

3. Use a meat mallet to smash the chicken thighs. Trim away any excess skin. Take a zipper-type plastic bag and add the chicken and the marinade. Shake the bag to ensure all the chicken pieces

have coated evenly with the marinade. Leave the bag to marinate for eight hours in the fridge.

4. Put the bottom and top plates on your outdoor grill and preheat using the med-high temperature setting.

5. Discard the marinade and transfer the chicken onto the heated grill.

6. Cook the chicken for about ten minutes. The juices will run clear by this time, and there will be no pinkish region in the center. Cut the chicken into strips and serve.

Chicken Lettuce Wraps From PF Chang's

Total Prep & Cooking Time: 45 minutes

Yields: Four Servings

Nutrition Facts: Calories: 269 | Carbs: 8g | Protein: 33g | Fat: 11g | Fiber: 2g

Ingredients:

For the Marinade:

- 2 tsp. soy sauce

- 2 tbsp. of sherry/red wine

- 2 tsp. cornstarch

- 2 tsp. water

Filling Ingredients for Lettuce Wraps:

- 1 tsp. ginger

- ½ cup minced shiitake mushrooms

- 8 oz. minced water chestnuts

- 8 oz. minced bamboo shoots

- 1 ½ lb. chicken breasts – boneless & skinless

- 5 tbsp. vegetable/peanut oil

- ½ cup minced garlic

- 6 oz. Chinese cellophane noodles

- ½ cup green onions

Cooking Sauce:

- 1 tsp. sugar

- 2 tbsp. water

- 1 tbsp. soy sauce

- 1 tsp. sesame oil

- 2 tbsp. oyster sauce

- 1 tbsp. Hoisin sauce

- 1 tbsp. sherry wine or red wine

- 2 tsp. cornstarch

- 1 head of iceberg lettuce-washed and left whole after taken off the head

Method:

1. Mince the veggies as desired.

2. Thoroughly mix the ingredients listed for the cooking sauce. Set aside for now.

3. In another mixing container, thoroughly mix the ingredients for the marinade. Add the chicken to this. Stir well and coat the chicken evenly.

4. Mix in one teaspoon of oil and let it rest for 15 minutes. On a medium-high flame, heat a large wok or a large skillet. While it gets heated, chop the chicken into small pieces. To the skillet or wok, add three tablespoons of oil. Stir fry the chicken in it for three to four minutes. Dump the mixture into a holding container, and place it to the side.

5. Add two tablespoons of oil to the same pan.

6. Stir fry the ginger, garlic, and onion, for a minute in the pan. Add the bamboo shoots, water chestnuts, and mushrooms. Toss to fry for two more minutes. Mix in the chicken to the pan, followed by the cooking sauce you have previously mixed. Cook until it is hot and thickened.

7. Cook the cellophane noodles, and break them apart. In the serving dish, cover the bottom with these noodles. Pour the chicken mixture on top of it. Serve with lettuce leaves.

Note: If you feel like making ahead of time, you can make the fillings and pop them into the fridge for two days. When you want to use them, all you need to do is microwave or heat them in a large skillet. If you have any leftovers, store them in the fridge for up to five days. Unfortunately, the leftover filling with lettuce will turn soggy, and this cannot be refrigerated.

Chicken Piccata at Olive Garden

Total Prep & Cooking Time: 30 minutes

Yields: Five servings

Nutrition Facts: Calories: 451 | Protein: 40g | Carbs: 6g | Fat: 29g | Fiber: 1g

Ingredients:

- 4 chicken breasts

- 1 small onion

- ¼ cup capers

- 10 - sun-dried tomatoes

- 1 tbsp. garlic

- 1 ½ cups chicken broth

- 3 tbsp. butter

- ⅓ cup heavy cream

- ½ of 1 lemon - juiced - about 2 tbsp.

- Black pepper & salt as desired

- For Frying: 4 tbsp. olive oil

Method:

1. Pound the chicken using a mallet until it's about a ¼-inch thickness and dust with salt and pepper.

2. Cook using the med-high temperature setting until golden and thoroughly cooked (approx. 5-8 min. per side.) Transfer the chicken to a holding container and set it to the side.

3. Slice the tomatoes into strips and mince the garlic. Use the same skillet to add the garlic, sun-dried tomatoes, and onions. Sauté until lightly browned (one to two minutes).

4. Rinse and drain the capers.

5. Whisk in the capers with the chicken broth and lemon juice. Take a minute to remove the tasty bits from the pan using a wooden spoon. Simmer the sauce using the med-low temperature setting to reduce in size by about half the volume (10-15 min.).

6. Once the sauce has thickened, remove the pan to a cool burner. Whisk in the butter. Once it's melted, mix in the cream and thoroughly warm the fixings (½ minute).

7. It's time to serve after you cover the breasts in the delicious sauce.

Notes: Use one to two tablespoons of the sun-dried tomato oil to replace part of the olive oil for a change of pace.

Easy Malibu Chicken at Sizzler Steak House

Total Prep & Cooking Time: 50 minutes

Yields: Four - Six Servings

Nutrition Facts - 4 servings: Calories: 696 | Protein: 46g | Carbs: 4g | Fat: 55g

Nutrition Facts - 6 servings: Calories: 464 | Protein: 31g | Carbs: 3g | Fat: 37g

Ingredients:

- 4 breasts of chicken (6 oz. each)

- Salt & black pepper

The Dipping Sauce:

- 3 tbsp. Dijon/ yellow mustard/combo if desired

- ½ cup mayonnaise

- 1-2 tbsp. keto-friendly powdered sugar **The Crumb Topping:**

- ¾ cup/36g - crushed pork rinds or panko crumbs

- ¾ cup /60g of grated parmesan cheese

- 2 tsp. granulated garlic

- ⅛ tsp. pepper

- 1 tsp. granulated onion

- ¼ tsp. salt **The Topping:**

- 8 or a total of 6 oz. - thinly sliced deli ham

- 4 slices or a total of 4 oz. - Swiss cheese

- Also Needed: 9 by 13-inch baking dish - glass is preferred

Method:

1. Warm the oven at 350 degrees Fahrenheit. Arrange the oven rack in the center-most position. Finely crush the pork rinds. You can use a rolling pin and crush them in a plastic bag or use a food processor.

2. Prepare the chicken by patting it dry. Sprinkle it using a portion of pepper and salt.

3. Mix the mustard, sweetener, and mayo in a mixing container.

4. Add ¼ cup of the mustard mixture to the plate with the chicken, saving the rest as the dipping sauce. Roll the chicken in the mix.

5. *Note*: You can also place the chicken in a bowl and mix it with the mustard mix and marinate it for up to one day. The chicken can also be cooked right away after you marinate it for ½ hour or so.

6. Combine the seasonings with the crushed pork rinds and parmesan. Sprinkle half of the crumb mixture into the baking container.

7. Add the chicken and the remainder of the crumb mixture over the chicken.

8. Bake it until the chicken is thoroughly cooked (30-40 min.).

9. Transfer the pan to the stovetop on a cool burner and add the ham and cheese. Pop the dish back into the oven. Serve after the cheese has melted.

Garlic Rosemary Chicken From Olive Garden

Total Prep & Cooking Time: 35 minutes

Yields: Four plates

Nutrition Fact: Calories: 336 | Carb: 4g | Protein: 48g | Fat: 13g | Fiber: 1g

Ingredients:

- 2 tbsp. - olive oil

- 3 cups - baby spinach

- 2 cups - mushrooms

- ½ tsp. of kosher salt

- 3 tbsp. of fresh rosemary

- 1 cup of chicken broth**

- 2 cloves of garlic

- 8 oz. - chicken breast

- ¼ tsp. - black pepper

- ¼ cup - dry white wine

Method:

1. Do the prep. Thinly slice the mushrooms. Mince the rosemary

54

and garlic. Trim the chicken to remove all bones and fatty skin.

2. Pour one (1) tablespoon of olive oil in a big skillet and warm it using a moderate flame. After the oil becomes hot, toss in the mushrooms and garlic. Sauté and brown them for about eight minutes and remove.

3. In the remaining oil, add the chicken breasts, pepper, rosemary, and salt to season. Prepare it for eight minutes per side until the golden brown color is seen and then set aside.

4. Keep the flame at medium, add the mushrooms back to the skillet and add the chicken broth and wine. Simmer for five minutes to reduce the broth and add the spinach leaves. Cook thoroughly until the leaves get wilted.

5. Shift the chicken pieces to the serving plate. Top with spinach leaves and mushroom to serve.

Notes: **Watch out for your health and use low-sodium chicken broth.

Instant Pot Chicken From General TSO's

Total Prep & Cooking Time: 24 minutes

Yields: Four Servings

Nutrition Facts: Calories: 427 | Protein: 35g | Carbs: 7g | Fats: 30g | Fiber: 2g

Ingredients: For

the Sauce:

- 1 tsp. sesame oil

- 2 tbsp. - no sugar added ketchup

- ½ tsp. ginger

- 5 tbsp. less-sodium soy sauce (gluten-free option - choose tamari)

- 1 tsp. chili paste

- 1 tsp. granular sweetener

- 3 garlic cloves

For the Chicken:

- ¼ tsp. each of pepper and salt

- 1 ½ lb. chicken thigh meat- boneless

- 2 egg whites

- 2 tbsp. - coconut oil

- ½ tsp. xanthan gum

- ½ cup chicken broth

- ½ cup almond flour

- Optional: Green onion and sesame seeds – for garnishing

Method:

1. Mince the ginger and garlic. In a bowl, mix the ingredients that are mentioned to make the sauce. Whisk them thoroughly and set aside.

2. Dice the chicken into small-sized pieces. Use pepper and salt for seasoning.

3. In two different bowls, place the egg whites and almond flour - separately. Rummage each chicken piece into the egg white first. Then coat with almond flour.

4. Use the sauté function to warm the coconut oil in an Instant pot.

5. Trim and add the chicken to it, and sauté it. If you are not able to do it in a single batch, do in multiple batches.

6. Deglaze the pot's bottom with the broth now. If small pieces are sticking at the bottom, get all of them with a spoon. Cover with

    the lid using the manual setting on the high mode, set for four minutes.

7. Release the pressure quickly and carefully. Using the back of the spoon is the right choice.

8. Thicken the sauce by whisking it with the xanthan gum. Cauliflower rice might be the perfect accompaniment for this recipe and keto-friendly too. You can garnish with green onion and sesame seeds if you prefer.

Note: In case you don't have an Instant Pot, try this in a slow cooker. For this, coat the chicken and brown it in a skillet. Add it to the slow cooker. Prepare the sauce and pour it over the chicken, followed by the broth. Leave the cooker covered in the low setting for four hours.

Keto Fried Chicken From KFC

Total Prep & Cooking Time: 26 minutes

Yields: Four Servings

Nutrition Facts: Calories: 440 | Protein: 30g | Carbs: 0 g| Fat: 24g

Ingredients:

- ½ cup heavy whipping cream

- 1 tbsp. - celery salt

- 3 tbsp. - paprika

- 1 tbsp. - garlic powder

- 2 lb. chicken thighs

- 1 tbsp. - freshly cracked black pepper

- ½ tbsp. - dried mustard

- 1 tbsp. - onion powder

- ½ tbsp. pink Himalayan salt

- 1 tbsp. - cayenne pepper

- 1 ½ cups pork rind breadcrumbs

Method:

1. Use a big mixing bowl. Trim the chicken - removing all bones and skin. Toss them in with heavy whipping cream. Place the chicken thighs, followed by the heavy whipping cream. Stir thoroughly. This is to ensure that all the pieces of chicken are coated well with the heavy whipping cream.

2. Set the chicken aside. It helps the chicken to soak in the whipping cream.

3. Use another mixing container to mix all of the spices and the pork rind breadcrumbs. Combine thoroughly.

4. Dip the chicken thighs that are soaked in the cream in the breadcrumb mixture. You need to ensure a thick and even coating is formed. Use a fork or tongs for this.

5. Start your Air Fryer to reach 390degrees Fahrenheit for 16 minutes.

6. If you choose, set the oven at 400 degrees Fahrenheit. Bake it on a baking sheet for 30-35 minutes.

7. In the basket of the Air Fryer, place how much it will hold. Do not overload the basket.

8. When done, remove from the Air Fryer and enjoy the delicious meat.

Summer Berry Chicken Salad From Wendy's

Total Prep & Cooking Time: 22 minutes

Yields: One Serving

Nutrition Facts: Calories: 315 | Carbs: 14g | Protein: 4g | Fat: 28g | Fiber: 4g

Ingredients:

- 1 chicken breast

- 4 oz. of lettuce mix

- ⅛ tsp. of salt

- ⅛ tsp. garlic powder

- ⅛ tsp. of ground black pepper

- ¼ tsp. dried parsley

- 2 tsp. vegetable oil

- ¼ cup blackberries- washed

- 1 tbsp. of feta cheese

- ¼ cup sliced strawberries

- 2 tbsp. blackberry vinaigrette

- 5-6 pieces of dried apple chips

Method:

1. Mix the salt, garlic powder, dried parsley, and pepper and season the chicken breast with this mixture.

2. Using medium heat, warm the oil in a small skillet. Wait till the oil starts smoking, and add the chicken. Cook each side of the chicken (5-7 min. each).

3. After this, remove the chicken from the skillet. Let the chicken rest for five minutes. Then, cut into small bite-sized pieces.

4. Add feta cheese, sliced strawberries, blackberries, salad, and apple chips to a large bowl. Finally, over these, add the chicken you have cut into bite-sized pieces. Generously add blackberry vinaigrette.

5. Add a few pecans after toasting them - making the salad creative and delicious.

Thai Chicken Pizza From California Pizza Kitchen

Total Prep & Cooking Time: 45 minutes

Yields: Four Servings

Nutrition Facts: Calories: 425 | Protein: 20.7g | Carbs: 28g | Fat: 35g | Fiber: 3.2g

Ingredients:

Spicy Peanut Sauce:

- 2 tbsp. sesame oil

- 8 drops stevia/sub for honey

- 2 tsp. - rice wine vinegar

- ¼ tsp. - dried red pepper flakes

- 1 tbsp. - oyster sauce

- ½ cup of keto-friendly peanut butter

- ½ tsp. - ground ginger

- ½ cup hoisin sauce

- 2 tbsp. water

For the Pizza:

- 1 tbsp. olive oil

- 2 chicken breasts

- 1 lb. pizza dough

- Cornmeal

- 2 cups - mozzarella cheese - shredded

- ½ cup bean sprouts

- 2 tbsp. chopped roasted peanuts

- 4 green onions

- ½ cup bean sprouts

- ⅓ cup carrots

- 2 tbsp. - cilantro

Method:

1. Shred the carrots and chop the cilantro. Diagonally sliver the onions and set them aside. Place a pizza stone in the oven. Set the temperature setting to 500 degrees Fahrenheit.

2. Prepare a saucepan, adding all the fixings for the peanut sauce. Gently boil just for a minute, and remove the pan from the stove.

3. Use a non-stick pan to warm the olive oil. Prepare the chicken by cutting it into ¾-inch cubes. Toss it into the heated pan to cook for about five minutes. Scoop the chicken into a mixing container, and toss with the peanut sauce. Use only half the peanut sauce for this process.

4. Make two halves of the dough. After dividing, make nine-inch rounds of each.

5. Use cornmeal to cover the pizza lightly. The pizza dough should be placed on the top of the round. Now use a quarter of the peanut sauce and pour it evenly on the dough.

6. Take ¾ cup of mozzarella cheese, and cover the sauce with it.

7. Place half of the chicken over the top, followed by the carrots, bean sprouts, and green onions.

8. Use the quarter cup of mozzarella cheese and half of the peanuts as the topping.

9. Place the pizza on the heated pizza stone. Bake the pizza for eight minutes or a maximum of ten minutes. The crust should be golden brown by then.

10. Dash the cilantro on the pizza after removing it from the oven. Repeat the same process of coating the pizza to place it in the oven for the other dough portion. After baking, sprinkle it as desired with cilantro. Your pizza is ready to serve.

3 Cheese Chicken Penne From Applebee's

Total Prep & Cooking Time: 45 minutes

Yields: Two Servings

Nutrition Facts: Calories: 662 | Protein: 22.25g | Carbs: 34g | Fat: 38g | Fiber: 2.4g

Ingredients:

- 2 chicken breasts

- ⅓ cup of Italian Salad Seasoning

- 15 oz. alfredo sauce

- 4 tomatoes

- 2-3 garlic cloves

- 1 tsp. basil

- 3 cups of penne pasta

- 8 oz. Italian cheese - shredded (or use parmesan/mozzarella or provolone)

- 6 tbsp. olive oil

Method:

1. Chop the chicken breasts. After chopping them, marinate the chicken pieces in the Italian dressing for thirty minutes.

2. Make the bruschetta. Chop the tomatoes and mince the garlic into a mixing container. Mix in the basil and toss, setting it aside for now.

3. In a pot of water, cook the penne.

4. Cook the chicken using the broiling or grilling method.

5. Take two bowls that can be used in a microwave oven. Toss the cooked pasta and divide it equally between the two bowls.

6. Over the pasta, pour the alfredo sauce. Repeat the procedure for the second microwavable bowl.

7. On it, add the chicken. It should form a layer over the pasta and sauce.

8. Microwave for three minutes. If you are using the previous chilled chicken, microwave till the cheese melts.

9. Serve the delicious dish with garlic bread.

CHAPTER 4: COPYCAT KETO FISH RECIPES FOR LUNCH

Bacon-Wrapped Tuna FromFoodpuckers

Total Prep & Cooking Time: 20 minutes

Yields: Two servings

Nutrition Facts: Calories: 699 | Carbs: 25g | Protein: 64g | Fat: 28g | Fiber: 0g

Ingredients:

- Salt & pepper

- 4 tbsp. honey

- ¼ cup Worcestershire sauce

- ½ cup soy sauce

- 4 bacon slices

- 16 oz. Tuna fillets

Method:

1. Take little portions of tuna and wrap them with the bacon slices. Secure the folding with the help of toothpicks. Put them on the grill.

2. Combine the honey with the Worcestershire sauce, soy sauce, and brush the mixture over the wrapped tunas.

3. Cook them until they are thoroughly cooked, i.e., until the tuna's color starts lightening, and the bacon starts sizzling.

4. Flip them over.

5. Cook until done. (Preferably medium-rare to medium).

6. Again brush the tuna with the sauce. Season with black pepper, and then serve.

Baked White Fish FromLuby's Cafeteria

Total Prep & Cooking Time: 30 minutes

Yields: Four servings

Nutrition Facts: Calories: 602 | Carbs: 12g | Protein: 36g | Fiber: 0g | Fat: 44g

Ingredients:

- 1 tsp. lemon pepper

- 1 cup mayonnaise

- ½ cup of all-purpose flour**

- Pepper & salt - as desired

- 24 oz. white fish (ex. - haddock or cod)

Method:

1. Warm the oven to reach 350 degrees Fahrenheit.

2. Blot the extra water from the fish with the help of paper towels.

3. Season both sides of the fish using pepper and salt.

4. Dredge the fish in flour, and shake off any excess flour.

5. Place the fish in a baking dish.

6. Evenly spread the mayonnaise all over the fish.

69

7. Top the mayonnaise with lemon pepper.

8. Pour half of one cup of water into the baking dish.

9. Bake the fish for about 15 minutes.

10. Heat the oven broiler and cook until the mayonnaise on the fish turns brown.

Note: **To make this dish keto-friendly, replace the regular flour with almond flour. This will prevent you from getting all those extra carbs. Whitefish have high phosphorus content that helps to keep your bones healthy. They contain vitamin B12 which contributes to the production of red blood cells. They also contain vitamin B6, B3, and some white fish also have vitamin B2. Due to their low-fat content, they also promote weight loss.

Batter-Dipped Fish From Captain Ds

Total Prep & Cooking Time: 20 minutes

Yields: Four servings

Nutrition Facts: Calories: 538 | Carbs: 15g | Protein: 45g | Fat: 41g | Fiber: 1g

Ingredients:

- Vegetable oil - as needed

- 2 lb. of cod or any other white fish

- 1 ½ cups of water

- ½ tsp. of cayenne pepper

- 2 tsp. of kosher salt

- 1 tbsp. of baking powder

- ½ cup cornstarch

- 1 ½ cups of regular flour

Method:

1. Use a medium-sized saucepan or a deep fryer.

2. Pour in oil and preheat to reach 350 degrees Fahrenheit.

3. Prepare a mixing container and add the cayenne pepper, salt, baking powder, cornstarch, and flour. Thoroughly mix.

4. Add a little water and whisk.

5. Continue whisking until the batter becomes foamy.

6. Pat dry the fish using a paper towel for removing any extra moisture. The process will make the batter stick to your fillets.

7. Dip the fish fillets in the batter. Coat the fillets thoroughly with the batter.

8. Start deep-frying the fish for about three to four minutes. Cook the fish until it gets a nice golden brown color. Hold your fish about halfway in the oil before dropping it altogether. This allows the crust to get a little cooked, thus preventing the fillets from sticking at the fryer's bottom.

9. Cook the pieces separately.

10. Drain the fillets of fish. Serve them hot.

Note: Whitefish have low-fat content and are rich in vitamins and minerals, making them an ideal dish for people who are conscious about their health. Whitefish also help you have a healthier heart and reduce the chances of a heart attack. A high level of triglycerides in your blood is responsible for heart attacks.

Whitefish lower the levels of triglycerides. People eating seafood have lower risks of developing dementia. The omega-3 fatty acids raise the serotonin level in your brain, helping you cope with depression. It strengthens your bones, thus relieving you from arthritis. They are observed to be good for skin as they reduce aging lines and give you a natural-looking healthy skin. Whitefish such as hake, coley, Pollack, sea bass, haddock, and cod are very beneficial for your health.

Country Fried Flounder From Red Lobster

Total Prep & Cooking Time: 30 minutes

Yields: Six servings

Nutrition Facts: Calories: 223 | Carbs: 18g | Protein: 31g | Fat: 22g | Fiber: 2g |

Ingredients:

- Oil (as needed)

- ½ tsp. of grounded black pepper

- ½ tsp. of paprika

- ½ tsp. salt

- 1 cup of cornmeal

- 2 lb. Flounder fillets

Method:

1. Skin the pieces of fish, and cut them into medium-sized slices.

2. Take a container and add the cornmeal, black pepper, paprika, and salt.

3. Turn on the oven. Pour oil into a skillet, and heat it over medium-high flame.

4. Rub the fillets in the cornmeal mixture, which was earlier prepared. Then put them in oil.

5. Cook the fillets for about two to three minutes until their color turns golden brown. Turn the fillet to the opposite side and cook for another two to three minutes. Check whether it is properly cooked or not with the help of a fork. If it flakes easily, then it is perfectly cooked.

6. Take the fish from the pan, put it over a paper towel, and drain it. Serve it hot.

7. You can also pair it up with coleslaw and tartar if you want.

Note: This can be an excellent and tasty option for health enthusiasts. Broiled, baked, or grilled Red Lobster dishes are the most preferred - rather than the battered and fried versions. Most of the dishes prepared from Red Lobster fish can provide an extremely nutritious meal. It has low-calorie content, which is why many people prefer it. It also has lowfat content, while comparatively, it has more protein content.

Fish is a rich source of selenium and copper. It also contains minerals, including zinc, phosphorus, and magnesium. It has vitamins like Vitamin E, vitamin B12, etc. It also contains omega-3 fatty acids. It is also seen that they can prevent you from the risks of developing thyroid diseases, anemia, and also prevents you from developing symptoms of depression.

Crawfish Bisque From Pappadeaux

Total Prep & Cooking Time: 1 hour 20 minutes

Yields: Four servings

Nutrition Facts: Calories: 415 | Carbs: 4g | Protein: 5g | Fat: 40g | Fiber: 0g

Ingredients:

- 2 tbsp. Brandy

- ¼ cup chopped tomatoes

- 1 ½ cups of whipping cream

- ½ tbsp. tomato paste

- ¼ cup green bell pepper

- ¼ cup onions

- 4 cups of water

- ⅛ tsp. of cayenne pepper

- ½ tsp. paprika

- 1 oz. of olive oil

- 1 ½ lb. of crawfish

Method:

1. Prep the veggies by chopping the bell pepper and onions.

2. Choose a big pot, pour water, and then boil the crawfish in it.

3. When done, drain the water and let the crawfish cool down a bit.

4. Separate the tail meat and keep it in the refrigerator. Keep the shells and head (though the only edible part of a crawfish is the tail meat. When you have crawfish bisque, you can use the whole portion of the crawfish and make a flavorful soup).

5. Heat the oven and warm a big saucepan to warm the oil.

6. Add the cayenne, paprika, and crawfish shells to the saucepan. Sauté them for five minutes, adding water as needed.

7. Wait for it to boil and adjust the temperature setting to low. Gently simmer for about ½ hour.

8. Take a separate pan and strain the liquid in it. Crush the shells and heads and extract all the remaining liquid, and add it to the liquid in the other pan, so that you will get a very flavorful broth. Get rid of the shells.

9. Heat the liquids in the pan, adding the cream, tomatoes, tomato paste, onions, and bell peppers. Simmer them for one hour, accompanied by frequent stirring.

10. Finally, add the crawfish meat and brandy and then again simmer for ten minutes. Serve it hot.

Note: Crawfish is rich in high-quality proteins, containing low-fat and carbohydrates. Crawfish are also rich in vitamin B and minerals (Phosphorous, Zinc, Iron, Magnesium, and Calcium).

Crispy Batter-Dipped Fish From Long John Silver's

Total Prep & Cooking Time: 20 minutes

Yields: Six servings

Nutrition Facts: Calories: 458 | Carbs: 18g | Protein: 31g| Fat: 19g| Fiber: 1g

Ingredients:

- Oil - preferably vegetable oil

- 16 oz. of club soda

- ¼ tsp. of ground black pepper

- ½ tsp. - paprika

- ½ tsp. of onion salt

- ½ tsp. - baking soda

- 2 tsp. - sugar

- ½ tsp. baking powder

- 2 tsp. - salt

- ¼ cup of cornstarch

- 2 cups of flour

- 2 lb. @ 3 oz. each of cod - cut into pieces

Method:

1. Prepare a heavy pot with eight cups of vegetable oil. Preheat up to 350 degrees Fahrenheit.

2. Prepare the batter. Grab a mixing container and add the ground black pepper, paprika, onion salt, baking soda, baking powder, salt, sugar, cornstarch, and flour. Add club soda (you can replace the club soda with beer for adding a better flavor), and start whisking. Don't stop until the batter reaches a foamy state.

3. Dip the fish fillets into the batter. Coat the pieces thoroughly and evenly and then drop them into the hot oil.

4. Fry the fish for two to three minutes till the batter becomes golden in color, and the fish rises to the top of the oil - floating.

5. Drain the fish fillets, and the dish is ready.

Fish Tacos From Rubio's

Total Prep & Cooking Time: 40 minutes

Yields: Six servings

Nutrition Facts: Calories: 404.4 | Carbs: 15.5g | Protein: 19.8g | Fat: 20.8g | Fiber: 9.5g

Ingredients:

- 12 gluten-free tortillas

- 12 pieces of cod @ 1 to 1 ½ oz. of each

- Pepper

- Garlic powder

- 1 cup of beer

- 1 cup of flour

- ½ cup of yogurt

- ½ cup of mayonnaise

- Oil

- ¼ tsp. pepper

- 1 ½ tsp. salt

- 2 jalapeno chilies

- 2 cilantro leaves

- ½ of 1 onion

- 6 seeded - ripe tomatoes

- 1 garlic clove

- Shredded cabbage

- Lime slices

Method:

1. Peel and dice the tomatoes. Chop and seed the chiles. Mince the onion and garlic. Remove the stems from the cilantro and chop. Whisk or sift the black/red ground pepper, garlic powder with flour.

2. Pour beer into the flour mixture. Continuously stir until it's thoroughly blended.

3. Wash the fish - by either dipping it into lightly salted cold water or by dipping it into the water with a few drops of lemon juice. Dry it completely.

4. Prepare the salsa. Take a pan, pour in oil, and add the garlic cloves, tomatoes, onions, cilantro leaves, jalapeno chilies, salt, and pepper. Nicely cook them and then keep them aside.

5. Pour vegetable oil into a skillet. Preheat up to 375 degrees Fahrenheit.

6. Dip the fish in batter. Evenly coat its entire surface, and then put it on the pan. Cook until the batter turns golden brown and becomes crispy.

7. Use a skillet, and slightly heat the corn tortillas until they are hot and soft.

8. Place one tortilla, add the fish fillet, layered with cabbage salsa and white sauce. Squeeze lime on top of it to give it a tangy flavor. Fold the tortilla. Serve.

Note: Cod is nutritious as well as flavorful. It is rich in vitamins, minerals, and protein. It has a low-fat content. It contains vitamin B, which improves your metabolism and helps in releasing energy from your food. It has vitamin B12, which is associated with red blood cell production and DNA. Vitamin B6 and niacin, present in this fish, help in many physicochemical processes in your body. It takes care of your heart health and promotes weight loss. Cod has low mercury content, unlike other fish.

Garlic Shrimp Scampi at Red Lobster

Total Prep & Cooking Time: 22-25 minutes

Yields: Four servings

Nutrition Facts: Calories: 284 | Protein: 38g | Carbs: 3g | Fat: 17g | Fiber: 0g

Ingredients Needed:

- 1 lb. Jumbo shrimp

- 1 tsp. McCormick's Montreal Chicken Seasoning

- Black pepper & salt

- 1 tsp. Italian seasoning

- 1 tsp. Olive oil

- 3 minced garlic clove

- 3 tbsp. of butter - microwaved for 15 seconds to soften

- Half of 1 lemon for juice

- 1 cup - Low-sugar dry white wine - Pinot Grigio Or vegetable/chicken broth

- ¼ cup Freshly grated parmesan cheese

- Optional: 1 tsp. red pepper flakes

- For the Garnish: Chopped parsley

Preparation Technique:

1. Peel and devein the shrimp. Give it a generous shake of salt, pepper, and chicken seasoning to your liking.

2. Add the oil and warm a skillet using the med-high temperature setting.

3. Toss the shrimp into the pan for three to four minutes. Once it turns pink, set it aside for now.

4. Mince and toss in the garlic to sauté until fragrant (1-2 min.).

5. Mix in and simmer the lemon juice, wine, Italian Seasoning, and pepper flakes (1-2 min.). Set to low for two more minutes.

6. Place the butter in the skillet to melt. Toss the shrimp back into the pan. Simmer for one to two minutes, and serve using parsley and parmesan cheese.

Honey Walnut Shrimp From Panda Express

Total Prep & Cooking Time: 25 minutes

Yields: Four servings

Nutrition Facts: Calories: 625 | Carbs: 26g | Protein: 29g | Fat: 27g | Fiber: 1g

Ingredients:

- 1 cup each:

  o Water - or as needed o

  Vegetable oil for frying

- ⅔ cup each: o White sugar o Cornstarch

- 4 egg whites

- ¼ cup of mayonnaise

- 2 tbsp. of honey***

- Optional: Scallions

- ½ cup of halved walnuts

- 1 lb. of jumbo shrimp (deveined and peeled)

- 1 tbsp. of keto-friendly *Sugar-free* condensed milk - sweetened (recipe chap. 7)

Method:

1. Devein and peel the shrimp. Prepare the condensed milk, as suggested in chapter seven.

2. Warm a saucepan on the stovetop. Pour the required quantity of water, add the walnuts and sugar as per the instructions. Let it boil - no more than two minutes. After that, transfer the nuts to a plate. Spread them out so that the water evaporates to dry.

3. Briskly beat/whisk the egg whites in a mixing container until they're foamy. Once they are done, whisk in the cornstarch - thoroughly mixing to incorporate.

4. Add the shrimp pieces to the whip, and with the help of a fork or a flipper, pick one shrimp at a time and drip them off to the whip one by one so that a thin coating is formed on the shrimp while you maintain its shape.

5. Warm a pan of oil to a temperature of 350 degrees Fahrenheit. Fry the shrimp pieces for approximately five minutes until they become light golden brown.

6. Prepare the sauce. Whisk the mayonnaise, condensed milk (sweetened), and chosen keto-friendly honey substitute in a small-sized mixing bowl and whisk to combine.

7. After the shrimp pieces are cooked, dip them one by one to the sauce and coat each of them using a spoon.

8. Place the coated shrimp pieces in a serving plate and crown them with candied walnuts.

9. Serve the dish with steamed rice, and you may even garnish with scallions (optional).

Note: ***The original recipe calls for honey. However, honey is not allowed on the keto diet. Therefore, you will need to substitute it with such as Maple Flavored Sugar-Free Monkfruit Syrup.

Tilapia Fillet From Paris Village

Total Prep & Cooking Time: 25 minutes

Yields: Four servings

Nutrition Facts: Calories: 480 | Carbs: 15g | Protein: 2g | Fat: 46g | Fiber: 2g

Ingredients:

- Salt & pepper - as desired

- 1 tsp. butter

- 2 apples

- 1 tsp. oil

- 1 tsp. white wine

- 2 cups heavy cream

- 2 sliced shallots

- 2 tsp. calvados wine

- 4 tilapia fillets

Method:

1. Warm a pan and add the butter. Add the apples and sauté them till they are caramelized.

2. Start seasoning on either side of the fish, and then sauté them in oil.

3. Use a saucepan, add white wine, calvados wine, and shallots. Cook them until they are reduced to half. Then add heavy cream.

4. Cook until the sauce is reduced and achieves creamy consistency.

5. The sauce needs to be seasoned and drained.

6. Take a dish, pour the sauce, place the fish, and then top it with the already prepared apple mixture.

Note: Tilapia has high-protein content. The calorie content is comparatively less; thus, it promotes weight loss. This fish is rich in minerals and vitamins. It has potassium, selenium, phosphorus, vitamin B12, niacin, etc.

Tuna Salad Sandwich From Panera Bread

Total Prep & Cooking Time: 5 minutes

Yields: Two servings

Nutrition Facts: Calories: 127 | Carbs: 1g | Protein: 19.9 g | Fat: 4.2g | Fiber: 0.1g

Ingredients:

- 4 slices of honey-wheat bread

- Salt & pepper

- ¾ tsp. of mustard

- 1 tsp. of sweet relish

- 1 ½ tsp. of mayonnaise

- 6 oz. canned tuna - drained

- Red onions - sliced

- Tomatoes - sliced

- Lettuce leaves

Method:

1. Grab a bowl. Add and mix the mustard, relish, mayonnaise, and tuna.

2. Put the mixture in the refrigerator for at least 15 minutes.

3. Place the fish on honey-wheat bread. Fill the dish with lettuce leaves, sliced onions, and tomatoes to serve.

Note: Tuna has an innumerable number of health benefits. It promotes heart health as it has omega-3 fatty acids and also helps to regulate your blood pressure. It improves your immune system as it is rich in vitamin C, selenium, manganese, and zinc. It contains vitamin B, which is known to improve your skin health. It improves your metabolism and provides energy. Lastly, it promotes weight loss because it is rich in essential nutrients and has low-fat content.

CHAPTER 5: COPYCAT KETO DINNER RECIPES

Angry Alfredo From Olive Garden

Total Prep & Cooking Time: 35 minutes

Yields: Four Servings

Nutrition Facts: Calories: 596 | Carbs: 2g | Protein: 21g | Fat: 56g | Fiber: 32g

Ingredients: For

the Sauce:

- ½ cup of parmesan cheese – freshly grated

- 4 oz. of butter

- ½ tsp. garlic powder

- 1 cup of heavy cream

- ¼ tsp. red pepper chili flakes

For the Chicken

- Salt & pepper

- 8 oz. breast of chicken

- 1 tbsp. olive oil

For the Topping:

- ½ cup of mozzarella cheese

Method:

1. Make the sauce. Warm a saucepan using the med-high heat setting to melt the butter. Be careful that the butter does not turn brown. Add the heavy cream, and wait till bubbles are formed. When bubbles begin to appear, add the cheese. Stir the ingredients frequently to ensure the sauce thickens to create a smooth consistency. Adjust the temperature to simmer on the stovetop. Add in the garlic powder and crushed pepper to the sauce.

2. Prepare the chicken. Use salt and pepper and season the chicken. You need a medium-sized skillet; a cast-iron skillet is preferred. Heat it over the med-high flame to warm two tablespoons of olive oil.

3. Cook the chicken for around five minutes or for a maximum of seven minutes. Once the edges turn white, this is the right time to flip the chicken breast. Keep cooking until the chicken is thoroughly cooked or for another five minutes or up to seven minutes.

4. Finish it. Set the oven to broil and preheat it. By now, the chicken is done. Allow it to rest and cool for some time (five minutes).

5. Dice the chicken into small chunks, so they are bite-sized. Mix the chicken with the Alfredo sauce. Place this into the casserole dish of one-quart size. Use mozzarella cheese as a topping, and place the casserole dish below the broiler. Wait till the cheese turns brown. When the cheese begins to turn brown, transfer it from the oven.

Note: The appetizer is served with sliced baguette bread - usually. If you want to keep it keto-friendly, use a low-carb bread or low-carb crackers. This also helps in checking the carbohydrates you consume with this appetizer accompaniment.

Beef Barbacoa at Chipotle - Slow-Cooked

otal Prep & Cooking Time: 4 hours 10 minutes

Yields: Nine Servings

Nutrition Facts: Calories: 242 | Protein: 32g | Carbs: 2g | Fat: 11g | Fiber: 1g

Ingredients:

- 2 medium chipotle chiles in adobo + 4 tsp. sauce

- 3 ½ cups beef/chicken broth

- 2 tbsp. apple cider vinegar

- 5 minced garlic cloves

- 2 tbsp. lime juice

- 2 tsp. cumin

- 2 whole bay leaves

- 1 tbsp. dried oregano

- 1 tsp. black pepper

- 2 tsp. sea salt

- Optional Ingredient: ½ tsp ground cloves

- 3 lb. chuck roast/Beef brisket

Method:

1. Trim the beef into two-inch chunks.

2. Combine the chipotle chiles with the sauce, broth, lime juice, garlic, vinegar, oregano, sea salt, cumin, ground cloves, and black pepper into a blender (all but the beef and bay leaves). Puree until smooth.

3. Toss the chunks of beef, the pureed mixture from the blender, and the whole bay leaves into the slow cooker.

4. Cook for four to six hours on high or eight to ten hours on low until the beef is tender and falling apart.

5. Trash the bay leaves, shred the meat using two forks, and stir into the juices.

6. Cover and allow the flavors mix for five to ten minutes. Use a slotted spoon to serve.

<u>Beef & Broccoli From PF Chang's</u>

Total Prep & Cooking Time: 25 minutes

Yields: Four Servings

Nutrition Facts: Calories: 255 | Protein: 28.2g | Carbs: 9.2g | Fat: 12.4g | Fiber: 2.4g

Ingredients:

- 1 lb. of beef - ex. sirloin, skirt steak, or flank steak

- 2-3 cloves garlic

- 1-2 heads broccoli - broken into florets (or pre-cut bagged)

- 2 pieces of ginger

- Ghee or olive oil

Optional to Garnish:

- Sesame seeds

- Chopped scallions **The Marinade:**

- 1 tbsp. + 2.5 tsp. sesame oil

- 1 tbsp. Red Boat Fish Sauce

- 4 tbsp. coconut aminos - divided

- ¼ tsp. - baking soda

- ½ tsp. sea salt

- 3 minced garlic cloves

- 1 tsp. - ginger

- ½ tsp. of black pepper - divided

- Optional: ¼ tsp. crushed red pepper

Method:

1. Combine the ingredients for the marinade and sauce (in two separate bowls) and set aside.

2. The Marinade: Two tablespoons of coconut aminos, ½ teaspoon of salt, one tablespoon of sesame oil, and ¼ teaspoon of baking soda.

3. The Sauce: Mix the stir fry sauce by combining two tablespoons coconut aminos, one tablespoon fish sauce, two teaspoons sesame oil, and pepper.

4. Slice the beef into ¼-inch thin slices and place in a pan with the marinade for at least 15 minutes.

5. Chop the broccoli (or take it out the bag if using pre-cut). Put it in a safe microwave bowl with two tablespoons of water and cover. Microwave for two to three minutes until it is tender but still has a crunch. Place it to the side for now.

6. Warm a skillet or wok using the med-high temperature setting along with one tablespoon olive oil or ghee. Mince and add the garlic, ginger, and salt. Sauté them for about 15 seconds.

7. Crank the temperature setting to high and add the marinated beef. Be sure to evenly distribute it and cook for around two minutes

(without moving it about too much) until the edges are dark – then flip and repeat.

8. Final Step: Add the sauce and stir-fry for about one minute. Mix in the broccoli.

9. Toss it further for another ½ minute and toss to serve.

Note: This recipe calls for coconut aminos, but you may substitute it with a gluten-free soy sauce or Tamari. However, you will need to use half the amount to achieve a more robust, saltier flavor.

Have you ever used Red Boat Fish Sauce before? It is a Vietnamese fish sauce that pro chefs often use to create that elusive "fifth flavorumami." It is made using black anchovy and sea salt with no added msg or preservatives. Each tablespoon of the sauce has 4 grams of protein, 15 calories, and -0- carbs and sugar. It is gluten-free and keto-friendly. Remember, this is the secret to the recipe: For this Keto Beef and Broccoli to be on point, you need to marinate the slices of beef for at least 15 minutes.

Chicken Salad From Chicken Salad Chick

Total Prep & Cooking Time: 40 minutes

Yields: Four Servings

Nutrition Facts: Calories: 430 | Carbs: 5g | Protein: 41g | Fat: 27g | Fiber: 1g

Ingredients:

- 32 oz. of low-sodium chicken stock

- ½ tsp. salt

- ½ cup of mayonnaise

- 1 ½ lb. chicken tenders

- 2 tbsp. - celery – finely minced

- ½ tsp. ground black pepper

- 2 tsp. dry ranch salad dressing mix

Method:

1. Poach the chicken in the chicken stock. Use an oversized pot to prepare the chicken stock and chicken tenders. Poach them for 15 minutes. You can extend by another five minutes to cook or until the chicken is thoroughly done - not pinkish.

2. The next step is to shred the chicken. You can use one of two methods for this. Choose a paddle attachment and shred with the stand mixer. The chicken tenders can also be shredded with two forks.

3. Take a bowl that is of medium-size. To this, add mayonnaise, dry Ranch dressing mix, celery, black pepper, and salt. Stir these well, and combine thoroughly. They should be blended well.

4. To this mixture, add the shredded chicken. Again mix thoroughly. You need to store this chicken salad for future use in an air-tight container.

5. If you want better results, you need to prepare the chicken salad a few hours before eating or serving it.

6. You can use this to serve with a sandwich or with bread lettuce. You can also serve it with any dish of your choice.

7. If you want to bring in more variety, add a tablespoon or two tablespoons of green bell pepper. You can place this in any container that does not let air escape. You can store in air-tight containers for a maximum of four days.

8. If you want to make this recipe gluten-free, you need to check the ingredients' labels. Some store-bought chicken stock contains gluten. Avoid them if you are on a gluten-free diet.

Chipotle Grill Gluten-Free Steak Bowl

Total Prep & Cooking Time: 25 minutes

Yields: Four Servings

Nutrition Facts: Calories: 620 | Protein: 33g | Net Carbs: 5.5g | Fat: 50g

Ingredients:

- 16 oz. skirt steak

- Black pepper & salt

- 1 homemade guacamole recipe

- 1 cup sour cream

- 1 handful fresh cilantro

- 4 oz. pepper jack cheese

- 1 splash Chipotle Tabasco Sauce

Method:

1. Prepare the steak with a dusting of pepper and salt. Warm a castiron skillet using the high-temperature setting. Once hot, add the steak to cook for three to four minutes per side. Let it rest on a plate while you prepare the guacamole.

2. Prepare the guacamole according to the below recipe.

3. Slice the steak against the grain into thin, bite-sized strips (4 portions).

4. Shred the pepper jack cheese using a cheese grater and sprinkle it over the steak.

5. Add about ¼ cup of guacamole to each portion, followed by ¼ cup of sour cream.

6. Splash each portion with sauce and fresh cilantro to serve.

Chipotle Guacamole Sauce

Total Prep & Cooking Time: 15 minutes

Yields: 1.5 cups

Nutrition Facts: Calories: 155 | Protein: 2g | Carbs: 2g | Fat: 14g

Ingredients:

- 2 ripe avocados

- 1 lime

- ¼ cup red onion

- 6 grape tomatoes

- 1 clove of garlic

- 1 tbsp. olive oil

- ⅛ tsp. black pepper

- ¼ tsp. salt

- Fresh cilantro

- Optional: ⅛ tsp. crushed red pepper

Method:

1. Do the prep. Juice the lime. Slice, remove the pit, and mash the avocados in a mixing container.

103

2. Dice the tomatoes and red onions. Add them to the avocado.

3. Mince the garlic clove and add the oil to combine.

4. Stir in the cilantro with the salt, pepper, crushed red pepper, and lime juice.

5. Thoroughly mix and serve with a steak bowl and a portion of pork rinds or low-carb crackers.

Chipotle Pork Carnitas From Chipotle

Total Prep & Cooking Time: 4 Hours 10 minutes

Yields: 12 Servings

Nutrition Facts: Calories: 223 | Carbs: 0g | Protein: 33g | Fat: 8g | Fiber: 0g

Ingredients:

- 2 tbsp. of sunflower oil

- 4 lb. pork roast

- 1 tsp. salt

- 1 cup of water

- 1 tsp. thyme

- 2 tsp. - juniper berries

- ½ tsp. ground black pepper

Method:

1. Set the temperature of your oven to 300 degrees Fahrenheit. This is to preheat the oven.

2. In the dutch oven, add sunflower oil in medium flame. Use salt to season the roast. Once the oil is heated, sauté the roast on all sides. This will take three minutes per side.

3. You will brown the roast a bit when you sauté this way. You need to add bay leaves, juniper berries, water, thyme, and ground black pepper to the Dutch oven.

4. Close the pan with the lid. Cook this in the oven for three to four hours. In the pot, you need to keep turning the roast frequently. Only then, the flavors will get into the roast, and it will incorporate the taste.

5. Take off the roast from the oven. Rest this for 20 minutes. Use two forks to pull the meat out of the pot.

6. Slow Cooker Directions: To a large skillet, add the sunflower oil. You can also add it to the dutch oven and warm it using medium heat. When the oil gets hot, sauté the roast.

7. Place the meat into the slow cooker and add water, ground black pepper, thyme, bay leaves, and juniper berries.

8. Cover the cooker with a lid. Cook the meat for three to four hours using medium heat throughout the process. While cooking, turn the roast once in an hour or once in 45 minutes or so. While you keep turning the roast less frequently, in this manner, you can ensure that the flavors get into the roast with ease.

9. If you want to use a pressure cooker for this recipe, it is notrecommended. Only a slow cooker will ensure that the meat

gets the perfect flavor. A fast cooking process using a pressure cooker will not give it a delicious flavor.

10. When you are choosing the pork, choose the cut that has marbling. Do not worry about the fat. You can always trim it.

11. If you do not prefer juniper berries, you can omit them. But the flavor would be altered when omitting juniper berries.

Note: For making the recipe keto-friendly, you can bring in avocado oil as a substitute to the sunflower oil.

Crawfish Etouffee From Magnolia Bar and Grill

Total Prep & Cooking Time: 40 minutes

Yields: Four Servings

Nutrition Facts: Calories: 237 | Protein: 3g | Carbs: 5g | Fat: 23g | Fiber: 0g

Ingredients:

- ½ cup of butter

- 1 tsp. flour

- ¼ tsp. cayenne pepper

- 1 lb. cleaned crawfish tails

- 2 thin slices of lemon

- 1 tbsp. green onion

- 1 tbsp. tomato paste

- 1 medium onion

- 1 tsp. salt

- 1 tbsp. parsley

Method:

1. To make the Etouffee, make use of a saucepan with a lid that tightly fits.

2. Use salt and pepper to season the crawfish tails. Keep the seasoned crawfish tails to the side.

3. Melt the butter in the pan. Finely chop and toss in the onions once the butter melts. Sauté the chopped onions over medium flame. Turn off the burner. Add the flour to the cooked onions. Stir and thoroughly combine them.

4. Then add ¾ cup of water - followed by lemon and tomato paste. Simmer and cook slowly for another 20 minutes. Keep adding water slowly, and less frequently.

5. When the sauce is cooked after 20 minutes, add the seasoned crawfish tails. Cover the saucepan with the lid. Cook again for eight more minutes.

6. Add salt and pepper, and check the seasoning for taste.

7. Now, add the parsley and green onion. Cook it for two more minutes. This goes well with steamed rice. Serve it hot.

Note: The recipe goes perfectly with white and brown rice. You can also serve it with spinach pasta, grits, and chopped and cooked cauliflower.

Hash-Brown Casserole From Cracker Barrel

Total Prep & Cooking Time: 1 hour

Yields: Ten Servings

Nutrition Facts: Calories: 488.4 | Carbs: 30.1g | Protein: 10.3g | Fat: 37.8g | Fiber: 2g

Ingredients:

- 1 pint of sour cream

- ½ cup margarine/butter - melted

- 1 lb. - frozen hash-browns

- 1 @ 10.25 oz. can cream of chicken soup

- ½ cup of onion

- 1 tsp. salt

- 2 cups of grated cheddar cheese

- ¼ tsp. pepper

Method:

1. Preheat the oven. Set the temperature at 350 degrees Fahrenheit. Use an 11 x 14 baking dish. Spray it with cooking spray.

2. Peel and chop the onion. Mix the margarine or butter, sour cream, frozen hash-browns, cream of chicken soup, onions, salt, pepper, and cheddar cheese. Combine them well, and transfer to the baking pan you have prepared.

3. Set a timer to bake for 45 minutes. You need to check if the top has become browned or done cooking at this stage.

Note: This comes handy when you have many people to feed or as a suitable recipe for brunch.

Southwestern Egg Rolls From Chilis

Total Prep & Cooking Time: 20 minutes

Yields: Six servings

Nutrition Facts: Calories: 502 | Carbs: 21g | Protein: 19g | Fat: 28g | Fiber: 3g

Ingredients:

Smoked Chicken Ingredients:

- 1 tsp. of olive/vegetable oil

- 8 oz. chicken breast

Egg Roll Filling:

- ¼ cup of green onions – minced

- ¼ cup of red bell peppers – minced

- 1 tbsp. of olive oil (Alternatively, vegetable oil can be used)

- ½ cup of frozen corn

- ¼ cup of frozen spinach - drained & thawed

- ½ cup of black beans from a can – drained & rinsed

- 1 tsp. of taco seasoning

- 8 - seven-inch flour tortillas

- 2 tsp. pickled jalapeno peppers - chopped

- ¾ cup of shredded jack cheese

Avocado Ranch Ingredients:

- ½ cup of milk

- ½ cup of mayonnaise

- ¼ cup of mashed fresh avocados (approximately half an avocado)

- 1 package Ranch dressing mix **Toppings:**

- 1 tbsp. chopped onions

- 2 tbsp. chopped tomatoes

Method:

1. Cook the breast of chicken. Start with seasoning the chicken with salt and pepper. Use a brush and apply the olive oil or vegetable oil on the chicken breast. On a medium-hot grill, grill the chicken.

2. Cook the chicken five to seven minutes on one side. When done, flip and cook the other side for another five to seven minutes. Cut the chicken into small pieces. Set it aside while you carry on with the next step.

3. Prepare the Egg Roll Filling: Sauté the red pepper. It should become tender. To this, add pickled jalapenos, black beans,

spinach, corn, and green onion. After adding these, add the taco seasoning. Heat the mixture thoroughly.

4. On the tortillas, place an equal amount of the filling. Then place an equal amount of chicken. Top them with cheese. Fold the ends, and roll the tortillas up. They should be rolled very tight to prevent the fillings from coming off. You can also use toothpicks to secure the tortillas from opening. Pin with these after folding.

5. Cook the egg rolls. Use a large pot and add about four inches of oil into the pot. Heat to reach a temperature of 350 degrees Fahrenheit. In the heated oil, deep fry the tortillas. They should turn golden brown. For this, it might take around seven to eight minutes. When they are golden brown, take off from the oil. Then keep them on a wire rack.

6. Prepare the Avocado Ranch Dressing. In a bowl mix, half a cup of mayonnaise, half a cup of buttermilk with the package of Ranch dressing mix. When thoroughly combined, add mashed avocado of a quarter cup to this mixture. In a blender, transfer this mixture. Blend in pulse option. The dipping sauce should become smooth, and when blended perfectly, stop pulsing.

Steak Gorgonzola-Alfredo From Olive Garden

Total Prep & Cooking Time: 1 hour

Yields: Four Servings

Nutrition Facts: Calories: 1584 | Carbs: 38g | Protein: 61g | Fat: 107g | Fiber: 5g

Ingredients:

Steak:

- 1 tbsp. of balsamic vinegar

- Salt & pepper

- 1 lb. of steak medallions

Alfredo:

- 2 cups of spinach

- 2 cups of heavy cream

- ¼ tsp. of nutmeg

- 1 cup of parmesan cheese

- Pepper & salt

- 1 lb. of fettuccine

- 1 stick or ¼ lb. unsalted butter

- 4 oz. of gorgonzola crumbles **Toppings:**

- ¼ cup of sun-dried tomatoes

- 4 tbsp. of balsamic glaze

- 2 oz. gorgonzola crumbles

Method:

1. On the steak medallions, apply salt and pepper. Place the steak medallions inside a Ziploc bag. Then add balsamic vinegar to it, seal and close the bag. Marinade the steak and let it stay for 30 minutes or leave up to four hours.

2. Prepare a large skillet using the medium-temperature setting on the stovetop. Add the steak medallions when the skillet becomes hot. It should reach the desired consistency. Based on the size of the steak pieces' thickness, the cooking can take time. Even after you stop cooking, it gets cooked. Cover the steaks with aluminum foil after placing them on a plate. You can cook the remaining elements, while this takes rest.

3. For the fettuccine pasta, start the water. Cook it as per the package's instructions till 'just shy' from being al dente. This is added to the sauce at a later stage and will be cooked then. When you are done with the pasta, drain the remaining water. You need to reserve a cup of water, which comes handy if the sauce becomes thicker.

4. In a large saucepan, mix butter and cream. Do this when the water is getting started for the pasta. Use a large saucepan or a wide

skillet for this. Heat in medium flame, and you should continue the process till the butter melts completely.

5. Bring the heat to medium-low. To the cream and butter mixture, add spinach and nutmeg. When the spinach wilts, you can stop cooking. This will take around five minutes.

6. Now add parmesan cheese to this, and season with salt and pepper. You should check for the taste. If you are using a salty cheese, you should refrain from adding salt after the parmesan is cooked.

7. Combine the sauce and the pasta. Toss quickly and ensure that the pasta gets coated evenly. Cook this now for two to three minutes to ensure the flavors are thoroughly combined. When you feel the sauce is thick, add a little pasta water, which helps loosen the sauce. You need to add little water at a time. If the sauce is thin, you can thicken it by cooking for some more time.

8. Remove the pasta from the heat after it has thoroughly cooked. Now, it is time to add the gorgonzola cheese. Toss thoroughly to mix everything thoroughly. When you add the cheese now, you can see little chunks are present and do not melt.

9. To serve, you need to place the pasta in separate bowls and plates. Place the steak medallions as topping on each bowl or plate. Add the balsamic glaze, followed by sundried tomatoes and gorgonzola crumbles used for garnishing.

CHAPTER 6: COPYCAT KETO SOUPS & SIDE DISHES

Soup Options

Baked Potato Soup From Bennigan's

Total Prep & Cooking Time: 6 hours 35 minutes

Yields: Ten Servings

Nutrition Facts: Calories: 212 | Protein: 7g | Fat: 18g | Carbs: 15g | Fiber: 2g

Ingredients:

- 4 cups chicken broth

- 2 onions - large-sized

- 2 onions (green & sliced)

- 3 tbsp. of butter

- $\frac{1}{8}$ tsp. of thyme (dried)

- 2 potatoes (medium-sized and diced after peeling)

- $\frac{1}{2}$ lb. of bacon (cooked, crumbled, and sliced)

- 2 tbsp. of (a.p.) flour

- 1 cup of Half-&-Half cream

- 2 cups of water - divided

- ¾ tsp. of pepper ● ½ tsp. each of:

  o Dried basil o

  Salt

- ½ cup of cheddar cheese - shredded

- 1 ½ cups of potato flakes - mashed

- Also Needed: 5-quart slow cooker

Method:

1. Take a large-sized skillet and add the butter to heat. Chop and sauté the onions to make them tender.

2. Mix flour in the skillet, gradually mixing in one cup of water. Heat the mixture to reach the boiling point. Make the mix a bit thickened by cooking for two minutes and frequently stirring for thorough mixing. Toss it into the cooker.

3. Cook and crumble the bacon and combine it with the potatoes, basil, chicken broth, potato flakes, thyme, pepper, and the cooker's leftover water.

4. Set a timer for the mixture at 6 to 8 hours using the low-setting after covering it. It will assist in making the potatoes tender.

5. Add the cream to the soup and heat it at the same time.

6. Use green onions and cheese to garnish the soup to serve.

Broccoli Cheddar Soup From Panera

Total Prep & Cooking Time: 40 minutes

Yields: Six Servings

Nutrition Facts: Calories: 589 | Carbs: 16g | Protein: 29g | Fat: 46g |
Fiber: 2g

Ingredients:

- ½ cup of white onions

- 29 oz. of low-sodium chicken broth – 2 cans

- 16 oz. American cheese

- 1 cup half-and-half

- 2 tbsp. butter

- 16 oz. chopped broccoli – frozen

- 1 cup of carrots – Julienne cut or shredded

- 2 tbsp. of all-purpose flour

- 8 oz. shredded cheddar cheese

- Salt and pepper - as desired

Method:

1. Prepare a large saucepan to melt the butter. Chop and mix in the onions. Stir and add the all-purpose flour. Stir and simmer for one minute. Add the half-and-half gradually. You should add only a quarter cup of half-and-half at a time.

2. Keep whisking, and continue the process until a thick and smooth consistency is reached. When you have whisked to integrate the half-and-half completely, add the broccoli. Then add the processed cheese.

3. When the cheese melts completely, add one cup of chicken broth. Stir less frequently, while you add the chicken broth slowly, one cup at a time. Mix and stir well to get a consistent texture. Now, add the carrots. Simmer it for ten minutes, and cook. After adding the cheddar cheese at this stage, cook for another ten minutes. Use salt and pepper for seasoning. Wait till the cheese melts completely. It should blend well with the soup. Now serve it hot.

Note: If you have leftover soup, you can refrigerate it. When you want to use it again, you can see that the soup has thickened. So, when reheating, add just a little milk. This helps in thinning of the soup.

<u>Chicken Enchilada Soup From Chili's</u>

Total Prep & Cooking Time: 6 hours 25 minutes

Yields: Eight Servings

Nutrition Facts: Calories: 125 | Protein: 14g | Fat: 9g | Carbs: 8.5g |

Fiber: 3g

Ingredients:

- 1 lb. chicken breast - boneless & skinless

- 3 garlic cloves

- 1 onion - medium-sized

- ⅓ cup of cilantro - minced

- 2 Anaheim pepper

- 8 oz. carton - chicken broth

- 2 tbsp. of tomato paste

- 1 tbsp. canola oil

- ½ tsp. of pepper

- 14.5 oz. can of Mexican tomatoes - diced and undrained

- 2 tsp. of chili powder

Optional:
- ½ to 1 tsp. of pepper sauce - chipotle hot

Optional Toppings:

- Sour cream

- Shredded cheddar cheese

- Crispy tortilla chips

- Also Needed: Five to six-quart slow cooker

Method:

1. Finely chop the onion, garlic, and peppers.

2. Use an oversized skillet and set the oven using the mediumtemperature setting. Then, pour the canola oil into the skillet and warm it.

3. Toss the onion and pepper in the skillet and sauté them for six to eight minutes to make them soft. Mix in the garlic and sauté it for one minute more.

4. Fold in the chicken breast and pepper mixture to the slow cooker. Combine the tomatoes, chicken broth, tomato paste, enchilada sauce, and seasoning into the mixture. Thoroughly mix. You can add pepper sauce as per your choice.

5. Use the low setting and cook the mixture for six to eight hours by covering the slow cooker with a lid to soften the chicken.

6. Take out the chicken from the slow cooker and use two forks to shred it.

7. Again, place the shredded chicken in the cooker and mix in the cilantro. Stir the mixture thoroughly and add the toppings according to your choice and serve it.

Note: Store the soup in a freezer-safe container and place it in the freezer; that is if you have any leftovers!

Chicken Gnocchi Soup From Olive Garden

Total Prep & Cooking Time: 60 minutes

Yields: Six Servings

Nutrition Facts: Calories: 446.3 | Protein: 20.9g | Fat: 25.1g | Carbs: 21.3g | Fiber: 3g

Ingredients:

- 2 stalks of celery

- 1 onion

- 4 cloves of garlic • 3 cups of chicken broth • ¼ cup each: o Butter o All-purpose flour

- 16 oz. pkg. - small-sized gnocchi

- 1 zucchini - large-sized

- 1 pint of half-a-half - fat-free

- 2 carrots - shredded

- 2 cups each:

  o Spinach - torn & fresh o Rotisserie chicken meat
- ½ red bell pepper - diced

- ¼ tsp. of nutmeg - freshly grated

- 1 tbsp. of olive oil - extra virgin

- ½ tsp. of ground thyme

- 1 cup of Half-and-Half

Add to Taste: One pinch - black pepper & salt

Method:

1. Use the medium temperature setting to heat a large-sized soup pot to melt and combine the butter and olive oil.

2. Chop and toss the onions, carrots, zucchini, garlic, bell pepper, and celery in the soup pot. Sauté them for 8 to 10 minutes and stir them frequently for thorough mixing to help the vegetables become tender.

3. Add flour to the mixture, and simmer for about two more minutes. Thoroughly stir as you continue coating the fixings.

4. Combine the chicken broth in the mixture of vegetables and simmer for nearly five minutes. Stir the mixture frequently to make a smooth soup to reach your desired consistency.

5. Simmer the mixture after pouring in both types of Half-andHalf. Cook it for about five minutes more to increase the thickness of the soup slightly.

6. Fold the gnocchi, chicken, and spinach into the soup.

7. Use black pepper, nutmeg, salt, and thyme for seasoning as desired.

8. If you want, you can mix in more chicken broth to adjust the thickness of the soup.

Note: Rotisserie chicken is advantageous to bring the best flavor. You can eliminate some vegetables to improve the taste of the soup as per your taste buds. You can use these vegetables for a side salad when you enjoy the soup.

Keto Chili at Wendy's

Total Prep & Cooking Time: 1 hour 45 minutes

Yields: Eight Servings

Nutrition Facts: Calories: 344 | Protein: 27g | Carbs: 11g | Fat: 21g | Fiber: 2g

Ingredients:

- 3 lb. ground beef @ 85/15

- 1 ½ cups - yellow onion

- ½ cup each of red and green bell pepper

- ⅔ cup of celery

- 1 cup of tomatoes

- 1 ½ cups tomato juice

- 15 oz. can crushed tomatoes in puree

- 1 ½ tsp. Worcestershire sauce

- 2 tsp. - granular erythritol - ex. Lakanto Golden

- 1 tsp. garlic powder

- 1 tsp. salt

- 1 tsp. cumin

- ½ tsp. oregano

- 3 tbsp. chili powder

- ½ tsp black pepper

Method:

1. Warm a soup pot (med-high heat) to brown the beef. Drain away the fat, leaving about two tablespoons.

2. Finely dice and toss in the bell peppers, onions, celery, and tomatoes.

3. Toss in the beef and simmer for 5 minutes using the med-high temperature setting.

4. Pour in the crushed tomatoes, tomato juice, seasonings, and sauce.

5. Place a top on the pot and simmer for 1.5 hours. Stir intermittently.

6. Before serving, transfer from the heat for ten minutes. Sprinkle with finely diced onions and a portion of shredded cheddar cheese for that Wendy's seal of approval!

Note - Each is a large version: Wendy's version; 23 carbs versus Keto version; 9 net carbs.

Sausage and Lentil Soup From Carrabba's

Total Prep & Cooking Time: 1 hour 45 minutes

Yields: Eight servings

Nutrition Facts: Calories: 353 | Protein: 18g | Fat: 22g | Carbs: 20g | Fiber: 7g

Ingredients:

- 48 oz. of (l.s.) chicken broth • 1 cup each:

  o White onions o

  Brown lentils

- 3 cloves of garlic

- 14.5 oz. canned tomatoes - diced

- ½ tsp. of salt

- 2 tbsp. of butter • ½ cup each: o Celery o Carrot

- 1 ½ tsp. of Italian seasoning

- 1 lb. of Italian sausage

Method:

1. Chop/mince and toss the carrots, celery, onions, and garlic in a large-sized pot and add olive oil. Sauté the mixture to make the onions transparent.

2. Mix in the sausage and cook the mixture until browned.

3. Drain the extra water if the sausage is lean.

4. Mix the chicken broth, diced tomatoes, brown lentils, and Italian seasoning in the pot. Simmer the mixture for nearly one hour and use a lid to cover the pot. You may add some extra water to the mix if the soup becomes too dry during the cooking procedure.

Note: You can replace butter by using olive oil.

Wisconsin Cheese Soup From Culver's

Total Prep & Cooking Time: 30 minutes

Yields: Eight Servings

Nutrition Facts: Calories: 292 | Protein: 14g | Fat: 21g | Carbs: 13g | Fiber: 1g

Ingredients:

- 4 cups of chicken broth - reduced- sodium

- 5 bacon stripes

- ¼ cup of all-purpose flour

- 2 cups of keto-friendly milk

- 3 of cubed Velveeta cheese

- ½ cup each -diced/grated of each:

  o Onion o Green pepper o Celery

  o Carrots o Olives - pimento-stuffed

  & sliced o ½ tsp. of pepper - coarsely

  ground

- Fresh parsley - minced

- Optional: Two tbsps. of sherry

Method:

1. Set the Dutch oven using the medium-temperature setting on the stovetop and fry the bacon until it's crispy. Transfer the bacon to a paper-lined platter using a slotted spoon.

2. Use the drippings to sauté the mixture of green pepper, celery, and onion until softened.

3. Combine the pepper and flour. Thoroughly stir them, gradually mixing in the milk and chicken broth into the mixture.

4. Cook and boil the mixture for one to two minutes until thickened. Add the carrots, olives, and cheese into the soup.

Also, include sherry in the mix as per your choice.

5. Cook the mixture and stir it thoroughly to melt the cheese.

6. Dice and sprinkle the prepared bacon and parsley over the soup before serving.

Notes: Alternately, set the oven at 350 degrees Fahrenheit and heat the oven before cooking. Use a jelly roll pan to place the bacon strips in a single layer and bake them to make them crispy. Use a paper towel to drain them after placing the stripes in a single layer and store them in the freezer.

Trim the ends and stem of parsley and keep them in a tumbler containing up to a half-inch height. It will help keep the parsley fresh for a maximum of one month - for later use. Otherwise, you can store parsley in the refrigerator.

Zuppa Toscana Soup at Olive Garden

Total Prep & Cooking Time: 40 minutes

Yields: Ten Servings

Nutrition Facts: Calories: 309 | Protein: 12g | Carbs: 5g | Fat: 24g |

Ingredients Needed:

- 1 lb. hot sausage - ground

- 3 garlic cloves

- 1 medium onion

- 1 tbsp. flour

- 6 russet potatoes

- 1 cup heavy cream

- 2 cartons chicken broth @ 32 oz. each

- 6 cups kale - torn pieces

Preparation Technique:

1. Crumble and toss the sausage into a large soup pot using the medium temperature setting. Once browning, dice/mince, and mix in the onion and garlic. After the onions are translucent, sprinkle using the flour and mix in the broth. Wait for it to boil.

2. Wash the potatoes and cut into halves lengthwise (¼ inch slices). Toss into the boiling pot and simmer until done (20 min.).

3. Set the heat to low. Pour the heavy cream and toss the kale into the pot. Simmer for about five minutes, occasionally stirring before serving.

Delicious Sides

Chips and Guacamole From Qdoba

Total Prep & Cooking Time: 10 minutes

Yields: Two servings

Nutrition Facts: Calories: 90 | Protein: 1g | Fat: 8g | Carbs: 6g | Fiber: 4g

Ingredients:

- 1 small-sized onion

- 1 garlic clove

- 1 to 2 tbsp. of lime juice

- 3 medium-sized ripe avocados

- ¼ to ½ tsp. of salt

- 1 tbsp. of freshly minced cilantro

Optional:

- ¼ cup of mayonnaise

- 2 medium-sized tomatoes

Method:

1. Finely dice the onion and garlic. Peel and dice the avocados into cubes.

2. Make a mixture with salt, garlic, and avocado after mashing them.

3. Remove the seeds and chop the tomatoes.

4. Combine the remaining ingredients into the mixture of avocado and stir it - mixing well.

Note: Avocado is enriched with a high degree of mono-saturated fat, named 'good fat.' It reduces the risk factors related to heart diseases and stroke by lowering the blood's cholesterol level. You can use delicious toppings to enjoy the chips and guacamole for tons of fun. You can include a unique flavor by using lime juice and lemon. Otherwise, you can use orange instead of lemon or lime juice to get the taste of orange in this recipe.

Chips and Queso From Qdoba

Total Prep & Cooking Time: 20 minutes

Yields: 24 Servings

Nutrition Facts: Calories: 95 | Protein: 5g | Fat: 7g | Carbs: 2g | Fiber: 0g

Ingredients:

- 1 cup of whole milk

- 1 medium-sized onion

- 4 oz. can of green chilis

- 2 cups of cheese - shredded - Monterey Jack

- 1-2 minced cloves of garlic ● 2 tbsp. each: ○ Butter ○ Cornstarch

- 2 ½ cups of shredded cheddar cheese

- Tortilla chips - as desired

Optional - As Desired:

- Jalapeno pepper

- Tomato

Method:

1. Chop/mince the garlic, onions, and chilis.

2. Warm a skillet using the medium-high temperature setting to warm the butter. Toss in and sauté the garlic and onion until softened.

3. Continue to sauté for about five minutes after adding chilies in the saucepan.

4. Use a small-sized bowl for mixing the milk and cornstarch to make a smooth mixture. Combine the fixings of the small-sized bowl in

the saucepan and heat it for one to two minutes to reach the boiling point. Cook and stir it to make a thickened mixture.

5. Lower the temperature setting and gradually add a small amount of cheese between two additions in melted condition.

6. Serve them immediately. Use tomato and sliced jalapeno or chopped tomatoes as toppings according to your choice.

Coleslaw From KFC

Total Prep & Cooking Time: 10 minutes

Yields: Six servings

Nutrition Facts: Calories: 283 | Protein: 1g | Fat: 24g | Carbs: 13g | Fiber: 2g

Ingredients:

- ¾ cup of mayonnaise

- ¼ tsp. of celery salt

- ¼ cup of sugar

- ½ tsp. of ground mustard

- 14 oz. pkg. of coleslaw mix

- ⅓ cup of sour cream

- ¾ tsp. of seasoned salt

Method:

1. Use a large-sized bowl for placing the coleslaw mix. Use a smallsized bowl to mix the remaining ingredients and stir the mixture frequently for mixing well.

2. Coat the mixture of the small-sized bowl by pouring over the large-sized bowl.

3. Keep it in the refrigerator before serving it.

Note: If you want to include more protein and less fat, you can use Greek yogurt replacing the sour cream. Mix ¼ cup of lemon juice or vinegar if your choice is for coleslaw tart. Otherwise, you can use a julienned apple to bring the taste of coleslaw tart.

Creamed Spinach From Boston Market

Total Prep & Cooking Time: 20 minutes

Yields: Six servings

Nutrition Facts: Calories: 186 | Protein: 5g | Fat: 14g | Carbs: 10g | Fiber: 2g

Ingredients:

- ½ cup of sour cream

- ¼ cup of water • 2 tbsp. each : o Onion o Butter

- 24 oz. of spinach (chopped, drained, and frozen)

- 1 tsp. of salt

The White Sauce:

- 4 tbsp. of flour

- 1 cup of keto-friendly milk of choice

- 3 tbsp. butter

- ¼ tsp. of salt

Method:

1. Use a saucepan to melt butter at the low-medium temperature setting. Make a creamy texture with flour and one-quarter teaspoon of salt and prepare a white sauce.

2. Maintain medium heat after adding a small amount of milk. Stir and whisk it frequently to make a smooth and thick mixture.

3. Chop and add the onions into a 2-quart saucepan. Cook it after setting the oven at medium heat and make sure the onions become transparent.

4. Mix the spinach and water in the pan. Keep the lid on the saucepan after lowering the temperature of the oven.

5. Stir the mixture frequently until the spinach is thoroughly cooked. Include one teaspoon of salt to get the perfect flavor.

6. Mix the sour cream and white sauce in the pan after the spinach has been thoroughly cooked. Simmer the mixture and stir it frequently to thoroughly blend all the ingredients.

Fried Cheese Curds From Culver's

Total Prep & Cooking Time: 20 minutes

Yields: Six servings

Nutrition Facts: Calories: 961 | Protein: 44g | Fat: 57g | Carbs: 27g | Fiber: 3g

Ingredients:

- 2 cups of breadcrumbs - Italian style

- 1 cup of all-purpose flour

- 4 eggs

- 16 oz. of cheese curds

- ¼ tsp. of salt

- 1 tbsp. of whole milk

- Vegetable oil - for frying

Method:

1. Use a shallow bowl and sift or whisk the flour and salt into it. Stir the mixture to evenly incorporate the salt.

2. Use another bowl and mix one tablespoon of milk with the eggs.

3. Beat the eggs correctly and use another container for placing the breadcrumbs.

4. Firstly, use flour to coat the cheese curds and then use eggs for coating. Lastly, use breadcrumbs for coating. It is essential to thoroughly and evenly coat the cheese curds.

5. Use a rimmed baking sheet to place the coated curds on the wire rack.

6. Then, place the cheese curds in the freezer to freeze them for 30 to 60 minutes.

7. Prepare a wire rack by placing a baking sheet or use a paper towel to line a plate.

8. Use a large-sized skillet or a pot and pour vegetable oil measuring up to 2 inches.

9. Set the oven at the medium-high flame and heat the oil over the flame.

10. Measure the temperature of 375 degrees Fahrenheit using a thermometer to ensure the perfect heating procedure.

11. Take care to drop the prepared cheese curds when you fry a few of them, avoiding crowding within the skillet.

12. Turn them once when you fry them for one minute - until they are golden brown in color after cooking them correctly.

13. Remove them from the frying pan using a slotted spoon. Serve them promptly for the best flavor results.

Mac and Cheese From KFC

Total Prep & Cooking Time: 2 hours 25 minutes

Yields: 16 Servings

Nutrition Facts: Calories: 388 | Protein: 17g | Fat: 28g | Carbs: 16g | Fiber: 0g

Ingredients:

- 3 cups of elbow macaroni - uncooked

- 3 large-sized eggs - lightly beaten

- 1 ¾ cups of milk - keto-friendly of choice

- 16 oz. pkg. of process cheese - cubed

- 12 oz. can of evaporated milk

- 2 cups of each - shredded cheese:

  o White cheddar   o

  Mexican cheese blend

- ¾ cup of butter - melted

- Also Needed: 5-quart slow cooker

Method:

1. Boil and drain the cooked macaroni as per the directions mentioned for making them al dente (8 min. approx.). Toss them

into the cooker. Combine the remaining ingredients in the cooker, and thoroughly stir the mixture.

2. Securely close the slow cooker's lid. Use the low-temperature setting (minimum of 160 degrees Fahrenheit). Stir once and continue cooking for 2-2 ½ hours.

3. Serve the mac and cheese piping hot.

CHAPTER 7: KETO COPYCAT DESSERTS

Chocolate Chip Cookie Dough Cheesecake From the Cheesecake Factory

Total Prep & Cooking Time: 2 Hours

Yields: 12 servings

Nutrition Facts: Calories: 801 | Carbs: 32g | Protein: 13g | Fat: 54g | Fiber: 1g **Ingredients:**

The Crust:

- 4 tbsp. melted butter

- ⅔ package of crushed Oreos **The Cheesecake:**

- 1 ½ cups of sugar

- 2 tsp. lemon juice

- Eggs - 6 whole & 2 yolks

- 2 ½ lb. of unchilled cream cheese - softened – cut into chunks of each one-inch splash⅓ cup of sour cream

- 2 tsp. of vanilla

- 1 tbsp. butter - melted

- ⅛ tsp. of salt

The Cookie Dough:

- 2 cups of flour

- ¾ cup of brown sugar

- 1 cup of chocolate chips

- ½ cup of butter

- 14 oz. can sweetened condensed milk (see recipe below)

- 1 tsp.vanilla

- Also Needed: 9-inch springform pan

Method:

1. The Cookie Dough: Beat the butter with the sugar and vanilla using an electric mixer. Slowly add the flour with the mixer set on low. The mixture will be dry.

2. Add milk and beat to combine. Fold in the chocolate chips and stir well.

3. Make balls of one-inch each. Keep in the freezer for forty-five minutes. Or leave till they are frozen completely.

4. The Crust: Preheat your oven to reach 325 degrees Fahrenheit.

   Toss the cookie crumbs with the butter. Add the mixture into the pan, press it, and bake for ten minutes. Cool completely.

5. The Cheesecake: Keep the oven heat at 500 degrees Fahrenheit. In an electric mixer, beat the cream for one minute on low. Scrape the sides. Add a three-quarter cup of sugar and salt. With the mixer on low, mix for a minute. Add the remaining sugar.

6. Scrape the sides, and add lemon juice, vanilla, and sour cream. Mix on low for a minute.

7. Thoroughly combine the egg yolks after mixing them. Now, add the two eggs at once, and beat for a minute. Now, add half of the frozen cookie dough balls. Stir to evenly distribute them.

8. Use one tablespoon of butter to brush on the top of the cookies. On the baking sheet, keep the springform pan. Pour the filling into the crust.

9. Bake for ten minutes. Reduce the temperature to 200 degrees Fahrenheit. Without opening the oven door. Bake again for ninety minutes.

10. Cool to loosen the sides. After cooling for two hours, wrap in plastic and refrigerate for three hours.

11. To remove from mold, wrap a warm kitchen towel. Then remove the sides and cut into twelve slices. Use whipped cream as a topping. Serve.

Keto-Friendly Sugar-Free Sweetened Condensed Milk

Total Prep & Cooking Time: 1 ½ hours - average

Yields: 15 servings

Nutrition Facts - per tbsp. : Calories: 165| Protein: 1g | Carbs: 1g | Fat: 18g | Fiber: 0g

Ingredients:

- ¾ cup erythritol-stevia blends/ex. swerve

- 20 oz. - heavy cream

- 2 oz. - unsalted butter.

Method:

- Toss each of the fixings into a saucepan using the mediumtemperature setting.

- Once boiling, while whisking, adjust the setting to a simmer.

- Simmer the mixture for ½ hour or until reduced by 3 ½ ounces.

- Add the condensed milk into a heatproof container. Pop it into the fridge to cool and thicken.

- The milk mixture is ready to use in about one hour. Make a double batch to use for other recipes.

Lemon Bread At Starbucks

Total Prep & Cooking Time: 1 hour 5 minutes

Yields: 15 servings

Nutrition Facts: Calories: 121 | Protein: g | Carbs: 3g | Fat: 10g | Fiber: 1g

Ingredients:

- 6 eggs

- 2 tbsp. unchilled cream cheese

- 9 tbsp. butter

- 1 tsp. vanilla

- 2 tbsp heavy whipping cream

- ½ tsp. of salt

- 2/3 cup Monkfruit Classic

- ½ cup + 2 tbsp. coconut flour

- 1 ½ tsp. baking powder

- 2 zest of 2 lemons (reserve 1 tsp. for the glaze)

- 4 tsp. fresh lemon juice

The Glaze:

- 2 tsp. freshly squeezed lemon juice

- 2 tbsp. Monkfruit Powder

- 1 tsp. lemon zest

- 1 splash - heavy whipping cream

Method:

1. Warm the oven to reach 325 degrees Fahrenheit. Prepare a bread pan using a layer of parchment baking paper.

2. Add the butter into a microwavable dish to melt. Let it cool.

3. Whisk the eggs, with the vanilla, heavy whipping cream, Monkfruit Classic, cream cheese, baking powder, and salt until combined.

4. Thoroughly mix in the coconut flour, melted butter, lemon zest, and juice to the mixture.

5. Scoop the batter into the prepared bread pan.

6. Bake it until the top of the bread is just beginning to brown and a toothpick inserted in the center comes out clean (55 min. to 1 hr.).

7. Prepare the glaze by combining the lemon juice with the Monkfruit Powder, lemon zest, and a splash of heavy whipping cream. Whisk until the glaze is creamy.

8. Empty the prepared glaze over the warm bread, spreading it out so that it covers the top and runs down the sides to serve.

Molten Chocolate Cake From Chili's

Total Prep & Cooking Time: 1 hour 55 minutes

Yields: 16 regular-sized cakes

Nutrition Facts: Calories: 723 | Carbs: 31g | Protein: 9g | Fat: 54g | Fiber: 4g

Ingredients:

The Molten Lava Cakes:

- Caramel sauce

- Chocolate shell ice-cream topping

- Vanilla ice-cream

- ½ cup sour cream

- ½ cup oil

- 1 cup of milk

- 3 eggs

- 1 box fudge cake mix **The Hot Fudge:**

- 1 pinch salt

- 4 tbsp. of unsalted butter

- 12 oz. of semi-sweet chocolate chips

- 1 tsp. vanilla extract

- 14 oz. of sweetened condensed milk (see the keto recipe)

The Magic Shell:

- ¼ cup of coconut oil

- 2 cups of chocolate chips

Method:

Prepare The Lava Cakes:

1. Use a large mixing container to add the cake mix, oil, milk, sour cream, and eggs. Thoroughly mix.

2. Use a large non-stick cupcake pan and evenly distribute the batter ¾ of the way full.

3. Bake at 350 degrees Fahrenheit (25-30 min.).

4. Take out the cakes and allow them to cool down.

5. Take a knife, start cutting a hole at the center, and don't go till the bottom.

6. Pour the hot fudge into the hole that you made in the cake. Then take the piece of cake that you earlier removed while cutting the whole, slice off its bottom circle, and put it on the top of the hot fudge just like a lid.

7. Wrap the cake pan using a plastic layer to freeze for about 30 minutes, or for up to two days.

8. Reheat the cakes, after taking them out from the freezer, in the microwave for about 30 seconds until it's nice and warm.

9. Top the cakes with caramel, ice cream, and the magic shell.

The Hot Fudge:

1. Warm a saucepan using the medium-temperature setting before adding all the fudge fixings to melt.

2. Stir continuously and wait for them to boil.

3. Continue boiling and stirring for about two minutes.

4. Transfer the pan to a cool burner and stir. Let it cool.

The Magic Shell:

1. Use a microwave-proof bowl to add the coconut oil and chocolate. Heat it at thirty-second intervals in the microwave - while frequently stirring - until it is melted.

2. Serve it over the cold ice-cream and allow it to harden.

Oatmeal Creme Pie From Little Debbie

Total Prep & Cooking Time: 25 minutes

Yields: 15 cookies

Nutrition Facts: Calories: 445 | Carbs: 25g | Protein: 4g | Fat: 28g | Fiber: 1g

Ingredients:

The Cookie Prep:

- 1 ½ cups of quick oats

- ¼ tsp. of cinnamon

- ½ tsp. of salt

- 1 tsp. of baking soda

- 1 ½ cups of flour

- 2 eggs

- 1 tsp. vanilla extract

- 1 tbsp. of molasses

- ½ cup granulated sugar

- ¾ cup of Swerve brown sugar - or another keto-friendly choice

- 1 cup margarine

The Filling:

- 1 tsp. vanilla

- ⅔ cup powdered sugar

- ¾ cup butter

- 7 oz. marshmallow fluff (see recipe below)

- ¼ tsp. salt

- 2 tsp. of hot water

Method:

1. Warm the oven temperature at 350 degrees Fahrenheit.

2. Make the cookies, take a large bowl and add eggs, vanilla, molasses, granulated sugar, brown sugar, and margarine. Beat.

3. Add cinnamon, baking soda, salt, and flour. Then mix the oats. Before adding the oats, make sure they are nicely processed into small particles, or else you may end up getting crumbs.Take a

parchment-lined cookie sheet. Drop the mixture by one tablespoon.

4. Bake them for about 8 to 10 minutes, until the edges turn brown. Check frequently to avoid overcooking.

5. Take out the cookies and allow them to cool down.

6. Then combine hot water and salt. Mix well.

7. Now for the filling, take a bowl and beat the marshmallow fluff with vanilla, powdered sugar, and butter. Add the salted water and mix well.

8. Take one cookie, spread the filling on top of it (you can use either an ice cream scoop or a piping bag to spread the filling evenly), and then put another cookie on top to serve!

Keto-Friendly Marshmallow Cream Fluff

Total Prep & Cooking Time: 15 minutes

Yields: 16 servings

Nutrition Facts: Calories: 14| Protein: 0.1g | Carbs: 0.4g | Fat: 1.4 g |
Fiber: 0.1g

Ingredients:

- ½ cup heavy whipping cream

- 1 pinch of pink salt

- ½ cup Swerve - confectioners-style

- 1 tsp. pure vanilla extract

- 1 tsp. xanthan gum

Method:

1. Prepare the fixings using a mixing container. You want it cold.

2. Have a hand mixer and spatula handy.

3. Add the Swerve or other powdered sweetener of choice.

4. Pour the heavy whipping cream over the sweetener.

5. Pour in the vanilla and pinch of salt, and whip with a mixer until fluffy like whipped cream.

6. Sprinkle a small portion of xanthan gum over at a time, folding and mixing with a spatula.

7. Continue sprinkling and folding until the mixture becomes sticky and thick.

8. Store in the fridge until needed.

Notes: Each tablespoon serving of this recipe has approx 0.1 grams net carbs according to the Carb Manager site. If you have a kitchen torch, this fluff will get nice and toasty!

Tiramisu From Olive Garden

Total Prep & Cooking Time: 45 minutes

Yields: Six servings

Nutrition Facts: Calories: 624 | Carbs: 34.6g | Protein: 6.8g | Fat: 38.9g | Fiber: 0g

Ingredients:

- Unsweetened cocoa powder

- 1 ½ cups of powdered (or finely granulated) sugar

- 1 ½ lb. of cream cheese

- 3 oz. of any liquor - preferably rum

- 3 oz. of strong black coffee or instant espresso

- 8-inch size sponge cake

Method:

1. Prepare the sponge cake. Slice it across the middle so that you get two even disks.

2. Use another container and blend in the liquor and coffee.

3. Separate the bottom half of the cake. Sprinkle the liquor coffee blend on top of it. Do it in abundance to get it strongly-flavored,

but be sure you don't end up saturating the cake so much that it collapses.

4. Use another container and start mixing the cream cheese with sugar. Continue beating till the sugar is thoroughly dissolved in the cream cheese. The mixture should become spreadable and light.

5. Evenly spread the cheese mixture on the cake's bottom disc (already layered with the coffee liquor mixture). Be sure that your cheese spread forms a thick layer and then keep this portion of the cake aside.)

6. Take the second portion of the cake and put it on the last half of the cake's cheese layer.

7. On top of this second layer of cake - sprinkle the coffee liquor mixture, and spread the cream cheese evenly on top of it, forming a thick layer.

8. Coat this cream cheese layer thoroughly with cocoa with the help of a wire strainer.

9. After completing its preparation, place the tiramisu inside the refrigerator for at least two hours. When you are ready to eat, cut, and serve.

Note: Instead of using cheese, you can use mascarpone. Either buy it or can also make it at your home. You can use any type of milk to make it. It's an enriched source of essential nutrients, including vitamin A, vitamin

B12, riboflavin, zinc, phosphorus, etc. It also contains highquality protein. It is a little expensive, but it can be found in various supermarkets.

To make mascarpone at your home, you will require some processed cream and one tablespoon of lemon juice or vinegar (to denature the milk). You will also need one thermometer, one double boiler, one strainer, and one cheesecloth.

Heat the cream, then add lemon juice to it, and then start whisking until it becomes thick. Then, cool it down and place it on the cheesecloth. Put it in the refrigerator for 24 hours. Take it out and strain the whey (you can use somewhere else). The remaining portion in the cheesecloth is the mascarpone.

Vanilla Bean Cheesecake From The Cheesecake Factory

Total Prep & Cooking Time: 12 Hours 25 minutes

Yields: 16 Servings

Nutrition Facts: Calories: 578 | Carbs: 39g | Protein: 6g | Fat: 45g

Ingredients:

The Crust

- 2 tbsp. of granulated sugar

- 6 tbsp. unsalted butter – melted

- 1 ⅔ cups crushed graham cracker crumbs

The Cheesecake

- 1 cup of granulated sugar

- 3 packs of cream cheese - softened

- 3 large eggs

- 2 vanilla beans - the seeds

- ⅓ cup of heavy cream

- ¾ cup of sour cream

The Mousse

- 1 ½ cups of heavy cream

- 1 ½ tbsp. of granulated sugar

- 6 oz. cream unchilled cheese - almost at room temperature

- 1 vanilla bean seed

- 7 oz. of white chocolate - roughly chopped

For Whipped Cream Topping

- 1 ½ tbsp. of granulated sugar

- ¾ cups of heavy cream

- Optional: Seeds of ½ vanilla bean

Method:

1. Crust: Warm the oven to reach 350 degrees Fahrenheit. Line the outsides of a springform pan, using a layer of fresh heavy-duty aluminum foil (18 x 18-inches).

2. In a mixing bowl, add sugar and graham crackers. Stir and mix well. Add butter and mix with a fork to aid in even moistening. Pour this into the springform pan. Bake it for ten minutes in the preheated oven. Transfer it to the countertop after ten minutes and place it on the wire rack to cool.

3. For the Filling: Bring down the oven temperature to 325 degrees Fahrenheit and boil four quarts of water in a large roasting pan.

4. Mix the cream cheese, seeds of two vanilla beans, and sugar with an electric hand mixer. When they are just smooth, add eggs one at a time, and mix. After adding each egg, beat, and combine. Combine after adding sour cream and heavy cream.

5. To release air bubbles, tap on the countertop about 30 times. Smooth into an even layer, after pouring the graham cracker crust over it—place cheesecake in a roasting pan, which you need to place in the oven. Up to half the cheesecake pan's height, you need to pour boiling water.

6. Bake for 65 minutes in the preheated oven. The cheesecake should be set, while the center should still be wiggly. Leave in the oven for ten minutes with the oven door closed. After ten minutes, transfer the pan on the wire rack for about ½ hour. Use foil for a tent. Refrigerate for eight hours. You can also leave this overnight.

7. For the Mousse: Melt the white chocolate in the microwave. Use a microwave-safe bowl, and do in 50% power in increments of thirty seconds. Melt until it's smooth and cool until it's lukewarm.

8. In a mixing bowl, whisk the heavy cream with an electric hand mixer. Add sugar and whip. Keep aside.

9. In another mixing bowl, whip the vanilla bean and cream cheese till they are smooth. To this, mix the white chocolate. Add half of the whipping cream and fold with a rubber spatula. There should be no streaks left out. Then, add the other half of the whipping cream.

10. Spread an even layer after pouring over the cheesecake. Use a foil to a tent, and store in the refrigerator for 1 ½ hours.

11. Whipped Topping: Whip heavy cream and vanilla seeds in a mixing bowl till you get soft peaks. Add sugar and whip again till there are stiff peaks. Spread the whipped cream with a knife. Keep for two hours before serving.

12. While serving, take off the foil from the pan. Pull the latch and remove the spring from the pan. Cut into slices. Garnish with raspberries and mint, if preferred.

CHAPTER 8: OTHER RESTAURANT FAVORITES

Avocado Egg Rolls From The Cheesecake Factory

Total Prep & Cooking Time: 30 minutes

Yields: 12 rolls

Nutrition Fact: Calories: 115 | Carb: 8g | Protein: 2g | Fat: 9g | Fiber: 4g

Ingredients:

The Dipping Sauce: ● 4 tsp.

of white vinegar ● ½ cup

each:

    o Honey substitute - ex. Lakanto Sugar-Free Monkfruit Syrup

    o Cashews (chopped) o Olive oil

● 1 tsp. each:

    o Balsamic vinegar o Ground

cumin o Freshly cracked black

pepper ● ¼ tsp. of powdered

saffron

● 1 cup fresh cilantro

● 2 chopped green onions

● 5 cloves of garlic

- 1 tbsp. of white sugar (granulated)

The Rolls:

- 3 avocados large

- 3 tbsp. of red onion - minced

- ¼ tsp. of salt

- 1 beaten egg

- 8 tbsp. of tomatoes (sun-dried), oil-packed & chopped

- 2 tbsp. of cilantro (freshly chopped)

- Wraps for rolling the egg

Method:

Avocado Rolls:

1. Do the prep. Peel, remove the pit and dice the avocados Mince the garlic and chop the cilantro and tomatoes.

2. Stir the avocados, tomatoes, cilantro, salt, and onion gently in a bowl.

3. Use a cutting board to place the egg rolls one by one. Brush the egg mixture on the wrapper edges. Spread the combination of avocado at the center evenly.

4. Start folding the rolls from the bottom corner and then gently rolling from the sides and then ultimately the top corner and seal it by pressing. Repeat the same with leftover wrappers too.

5. Deep fry the wrappers in oil over moderate heat. Submerge rolls in oil for better frying. Fry in batches with each batch for four minutes until they become golden brown.

6. Place them on the paper towels and then serve on a plate. Serve with dipping sauce.

The Sauce:

1. Mix the saffron powder, honey, and vinegar in a microwave-safe bowl and microwave for about one minute and stir it again. Keep it away.

2. Add the honey mixture and the remaining ingredients for preparing the sauce using a blender and then process.

3. Pour the sauce in a bowl, and you may make it thin by stirring in olive oil. Keep in a refrigerator until it is used.

Note: Avocado has its name for increasing the levels of good cholesterols (HDL). Other uses include promoting healthy hair growth, stimulates the flow of menstruation, reduces diarrhea, helps reduce toothache, and sclerosis.

Big Mac Salad From McDonald's

Total Prep Time: 30 minutes

Yields: Four plates

Nutrition Fact: Calories: 511 | Carb: 4g | Protein: 36g | Fat: 34g | Fiber: 3g

Ingredients:

- 1 lb. of ground beef

- 6 cups of iceberg lettuce - torn

- 1 cup of salad croutons

- 1 small onion

- Salad dressing

- 2 tsp. of Montreal steak seasoning

- 2 cups of cheddar cheese - shredded

- 1 medium-sized tomato

- ½ cup of sliced dill pickle

Method:

1. In a large-sized bowl, thoroughly combine the steak seasoning and beef. Shape it into patties of ½-inch.

172

2. Grill the burgers over moderate heat for about four minutes with the lid *on*. Cook both sides until the internal temperature reaches 160 degrees Fahrenheit.

3. Thinly slice the onion and chop the tomato.

4. Toss the salad fixings and burgers, croutons, onions, pickles, lettuce, cheese, and tomato. Serve.

In & Out Restaurant Burgers

Total Prep & Cooking Time: 20 minutes

Yields: Five Servings

Nutrition Facts: Calories: 371| Protein: 34g | Carbs: 3g | Fat: 24g | Fiber: 0g **Ingredients:**

The Burgers:

- 1 lb. - 80/20 preferred - ground beef

- Black pepper and salt

- 4 slices of yellow American cheese

The Sauce:

- 1/3 cup Mayonnaise - regular or avocado

- 1 tsp. mustard

- 1 tbsp. sugar-free ketchup/1 tsp. organic tomato paste

- 1-2 tsp. pickle juice

- 2 tbsp. diced pickles

- ½ tsp. salt

- ½ tsp. garlic powder

- ½ tsp. paprika **The Toppings:**

174

- Iceberg lettuce as a bun

- Sliced tomato

- Pickles

- ½ thinly sliced yellow onion

Method:

1. Prepare the sauce. Use a small mixing container to combine the mayo, ketchup, diced pickles, pickle juice, mustard, and spices. Thoroughly combine.

2. Prepare the burger patties (about ¼ cup each) and roll into a meatball. Repeat until you have ten meatballs. Sprinkle them using a bit of cracked black pepper and salt.

3. Warm a cast-iron skillet or griddle using the high-temperature setting. Add a small portion of oil to the pan if necessary. Place two meatballs onto the griddle or pan and use a wide spatula and press down.

4. Baste the top in mustard before flipping for extra flavor if desired. As the edges are browned, flip them over and add a slice of cheese on one burger patty and stack the second patty over it.

5. To assemble the patty, begin with the bun (lettuce) and add sliced onion, the double-stacked burger, tomato, pickles, and the sauce. Cover with the second lettuce bun and serve.

Note: The nutritional facts list only the sauce and burger. You will need to add additions, including onions, lettuce, tomatoes, etc. The traditional 'In & Out burger caramelizes the onions.

Smoked Mozzarella Founduta From Olive Garden

Total Prep & Cooking Time: 25 minutes

Yields: Eight pieces

Nutrition Fact: Calories: 275 | Carbs: 21.8g | Protein: 27.2g | Fat: 30.6g | Fiber: 1.1g

Ingredients:

- 1 loaf of Italian bread - sliced into slices of ¼-inch

- 1 tsp. of thyme

- ¼ tsp. of cayenne pepper

- 3 cups of shredded provolone cheese - smoked or normal • 3 tbsp. grated of each: o Romano cheese o Parmesan cheese

- 1 cup of sour cream

- ½ tsp. of crushed flakes of red pepper

- 3 cups of mozzarella cheese - shredded - normal or smoked

- Also Needed: 8x10 baking tray/dish or 8 ramekins

To Serve:

- Freshly chopped parsley

- 8 tsp. of freshly diced tomatoes

Method:

1. Warm the oven at 450 degrees Fahrenheit.

2. Arrange the flat surfaces of the bread onto a baking sheet and cover them using foil. Set the preparation aside until they are needed.

3. Use a bowl to combine the four types of cheese, thyme, cayenne pepper, red pepper, and the sour cream.

4. Spray the pan/ramekins using a spritz of cooking oil spray. Transfer the mixture to it using a spatula. If using ramekins, fill each cup with the mixture only up to its half. On a baking sheet, add the mixture to the bowl. Place the mix of cheese to form an even surface on each of the cups.

To Bake:

1. According to your serving style, place either the baking sheet/casserole dish at the oven's center rack.

2. Place the baking tray, which has the bread in it covered after about five minutes, on the oven's upper rack. Bake for another five minutes and then remove the fonduta and the bread from the oven.

To Serve:

1. Place the diced tomato on the casserole dish and arrange the fonduta centered with parsley.

2. If using bowls, divide the two of these evenly among them and arrange the bread slices around bowls and serve.

Note: An essential ingredient of this recipe is mozzarella, which has many health benefits. It is a good source of biotin, which is not stored easily by the body and will also meet your nutritional needs. It is an excellent riboflavin source, which can benefit the body by fighting against problems like anemia and migraine attacks. It helps to restore the fat-soluble vitamins and zinc. It also helps to make your bones stronger and is known to be the powerhouse of protein. Plus, you feel energetic and are increasing your muscle strength.

Loaded Potato Skins From TGI Fridays

Total Prep & Cooking Time: 30 minutes

Yields: Eight servings

Nutrition Fact: Calories: 350 | Carb: 2g | Protein: 12g | Fat: 19g | Fiber: 4g

Ingredients:

- 4 large baked potatoes

- 1 tbsp. of parmesan cheese (grated) ☐ ¼ tsp. each: o Paprika o

  Garlic powder

- 8 strips of bacon

- ½ cup of sour cream

- 3 tbsp. of olive/another keto-friendly oil

- ½ tsp. of salt

- ⅛ tsp. of pepper

- 1 ½ cups of shredded cheddar cheese

- 4 sliced green onions

Method:

1. Warm the oven temperature at 475 degrees Fahrenheit.

2. Scoop the pulp from the potatoes after cutting them into halves -
   lengthwise. Leave 'only' ¼ of the pulp in the skin and store the
   rest for use later.

3. Lightly grease a baking sheet and arrange the skins on it.

4. Combine the parmesan cheese, garlic powder, pepper, oil, salt, and
   paprika. With this mixture, brush the sides of the skins.

5. Bake each side for seven minutes, so they become crispy. You can also bake the bacon in the oven or skillet until it's crispy. Sprinkle cheddar cheese and bacon bits over the potato skins.

6. Bake for another two minutes to melt the cheese. Garnish with onions and cream to serve.

Note: ***Canola oil contains a high amount of mono-saturated fat, which is considered extremely good for your health. It has been found to lower cholesterol levels in the blood. They are also low in saturated fat, which can increase cholesterol in the blood. Olive oil can be mixed with this recipe as it also has the same properties as having healthy fat.

However, keto says it is a 'no-go.' They contain high amounts of polyunsaturated fats.

Instead, choose a keto-friendly option as mentioned previously;

- Coconut oil

- Extra-virgin olive oil

- Avocado oil

- MCT oil

- Sesame oil

- Palm oil

CHAPTER 9: OTHER RESTAURANT BEVERAGE FAVORITES

Frappuccino At Starbucks

Total Prep & Cooking Time: 5 minutes

Yields: Six Servings

Nutrition Facts: Calories: 182 | Protein: 1g | Carbs: 1.2g | Fat: 14.7g | Fiber: 0.6g

Ingredients:

- 1 cup strong cooled coffee

- 1 cup heavy cream

- 1 ½ tbsp. stevia erythritol blend

- ⅓ cups of ice

- Optional Garnish: Whipped cream & additional low-carb caramel sauce

Method:

1. Use an electric blender with ice crushing capacity, and combine each of the fixings. Blend until smooth - as a slushie.

2. Pour the mixture into chilled glasses and serve with whipped cream and low-carb caramel sauce to your liking.

Iced Skinny Vanilla Latte & Frappuccino At Starbucks

Total Prep & Cooking Time: 5 minutes

Yields: Six Servings

Nutrition Facts: Calories: 79 | Protein: 0g | Carbs: 0g | Fat: 8g | Fiber: 0g

Ingredients:

The Concentrate:

- 1 ½ cups almond milk

- ½ cup heavy cream

- 1 cup very very strong coffee (about double the regular amount of grounds)

- ½ cup - natural sweetener (below recipe)

- 1 tsp. vanilla

Method:

1. Make the Concentrate: Toss all of the components and thoroughly mix them.

2. To Make an Iced Latte:

3. 1 part concentrate = 1 to 1.5 parts almond milk + coffee ice cubes (frozen coffee in an ice cube tray)

4. Latte Example: 6 oz. concentrate + 8 oz. of almond milk over frozen coffee ice cubes

5. To Make a Frappuccino:

6. Blend 1 part concentrate, coffee ice cubes and regular ice cubes, a pinch of xanthan gum, and ½ part almond milk.

7. Frappuccino Example: 8 oz. concentrate + 4 oz. almond milk blended with 6 coffee ice cubes, 6 regular ice cubes, and a pinch of xanthan gum.

Natural Keto-Friendly Sugar Sweetener

Total Prep & Cooking Time: 5 minutes

Yields: 64 tablespoons

Nutrition Facts: Calories: 1 | Carbs: 0.1g | Fiber: 0.1g **Ingredients:**

- 12 oz. or 1 ½ cups + 2 tbsp. erythritol

- 16 oz. or 2 cups + 2 tbsp. xylitol

- 2 tsp. pure stevia extract

Method:

1. Granular Sweetener: For baking and candy making, you can just mix the ingredients together by hand.

2. Powdered Sweetener: Process the ingredients in the food processor for a few minutes if you are planning on using it in chocolate, beverages, or icing.

Orange Julius by Dairy Queen

Total Prep & Cooking Time: 5 minutes

Yields: Two Servings

Nutrition Facts: Calories: 367 | Protein: 2g | Carbs: 15.5g | Fat: 42g | Fiber: 0g

Ingredients:

- 2/3 cup heavy whipping cream

- 3 tbsp./as desired of confectioners erythritol

- 2 to 3 oz. cream cheese

- 1 ½ tsp. pure orange extract

- 1 ½ tsp. lemon juice

- 2 to 2 ½ cups crushed ice

Optional Ingredients:

- Food coloring

- To Garnish: Orange slice

Method:

1. Add heavy whipping cream to a blender. Blend for a minute or so until the cream has churned into a thick whipped cream.

2. Add the cream cheese, erythritol, pure orange extract, lemon juice, food coloring , and crushed ice. Using crushed ice vs. ice cubes helps the shake come together quickly. Blend until even and smooth, about a minute.

3. Pour into one large or two small glasses. Garnish with an orange slice if desired.

Notes: Dairy Queen bought the Orange Julius chain in 1987 and began adding it to its small Treat Center locations the following year.

Peppermint Mocha at Starbucks

Total Prep & Cooking Time: 3 minutes

Yields: One Serving

Nutrition Facts: Calories: 197 | Protein: 1g | Carbs: 5.2g | Fat: 19g | Fiber: 2.8g

Ingredients:

- 2 tbsp. heavy whipping cream

- 1 cup unsweetened (carton only) coconut/almond milk

- 4 oz. brewed blonde roast coffee

- 1 tbsp. Dutch-process cocoa powder

- 3 tbsp. Swerve Confectioners

- 1 tbsp. Perfect Keto Chocolate MCT Oil Powder

- ¼ tsp. or as desired - peppermint extract

- 100% cacao chocolate or another keto-friendly chocolate shavings

- Optional: Keto-friendly whipped cream

Method:

1. Combine all of the fixings (omit the peppermint extract) using an electric whisk to make the process much simpler. Place them

188

in a pan to warm using the medium-temperature setting.

2. Warm the mixture to your desired temperature (2 min.), turn off the heat, add the peppermint extract, and mix it again.

3. Pour the treat into a glass, top it off using your favorite ketofriendly whipped cream and/or chocolate shavings to serve.

Shamrock Shake From McDonald's

Total Prep & Cooking Time: 6 minutes

Yields: Two glasses

Nutrition Fact: Calories: 330 | Carb: 15g | Protein: 7g | Fat: 17g | Fiber: 0g

Ingredients:

- 2 cups of ice cream (vanilla)

- 10 drops of food coloring (green)

- Whipped cream and cherries

- ¾ cup of whole milk

- ¼ tsp. of mint extract

Method:

1. Switch on the blender and place the milk, mint extract, food coloring, and ice cream in it.

2. Blend the ingredients until they become smooth.

3. Pour them in the tall glasses (two) and crown each of them with cream, cherries, and sprinkles to serve.

Wendy's Inspired Keto Chocolate Frosty

Total Prep & Cooking Time: 10 minutes

Yields: Four Servings

Nutrition Facts: Calories: 241 | Protein: 3g | Carbs: 4g | Fat: 25 g | Fiber: 1g

Ingredients Needed:

- 1 cup heavy whipping cream

- 1 tbsp. almond butter

- 2 tbsp. unsweetened cocoa powder

- 5-10 drops - to taste of Stevia

- 1 tsp. vanilla extract

Preparation Technique:

1. Combine all of the fixings using an electric mixer until it forms stiff peaks.

2. Pop the mixture into the freezer for 30 minutes to one hour or until it's barely frozen.

3. Dump the 'frosty' mixture into a plastic freezer bag.

4. Make a piping bag by snipping the corner from the bag. Pipe the frosty into the chilled glasses.

Notes: Look at the comparisons; they show positive results:

a) Wendy's Version (small): 54 carbs

b) Keto version (small): 3 net carbs

CONCLUSION

I hope you have found many new recipes to serve your family in your copy of Keto Copycat Recipes. I hope it was informative and provided you with all of the tools you need to achieve your goals - whatever they may be.

The next step is to head to the market to fill your kitchen with all of the essentials.

Gather all of the fixings and start your next new masterpiece.

Hopefully, by now, you must have realized how easy it is to cook your own meals at home. This book has provided you with keto-friendly recipes from different restaurants. This will also help you save some money since making those same dishes at home will be way more costeffective than dining out to the restaurant for lunch or dinner.

Whether you want to have cheesecakes for dessert or a burrito bowl for lunch, you can make them in the comfort of your own home with healthy ingredients. The recipes mentioned in this book are great for anyone looking for restaurant-style food but more healthy. If you are considering hosting a party in your house, this recipe book will significantly help. I wanted to motivate everyone to cook their favorite dishes at home through this book. My only aim was to show you how easy it is. I hope this book has successfully taught you some tricks in making the best homemade restaurant-style meals.

As a little bonus, do you love Girl Scout cookies? If you enjoy Tagalongs, take a look at this keto-friendly recipe!

Tagalongs - Peanut Butter Patties

Total Prep & Cooking Time: 1 ½ hours - + minutes

Yields: 36 cookies @ 2 per serving

Nutrition Facts: Calories: | Protein: g | Carbs: g | Fat: g | Fiber: g

Ingredients:

The Shortbread Cookies:

- 2 cups almond flour

- ½ cup Swerve Sweetener

- 1 tsp. baking powder

- 1 pinch of salt

- 1 large egg

- 2 tbsp. melted butter

- 1 tsp. vanilla extract

The Filling:

- 1 cup Keto-friendly creamy peanut butter (see below)

- 2 tbsp butter

- 1/4 cup confectioner's Swerve Sweetener **The Chocolate**

Coating:

- 7 oz. of 85 to 90% dark chocolate - chopped

- 1 tbsp. butter

Method:

The Shortbread Cookies:

1. Warm the oven at 300 degrees Fahrenheit. Cover two cookie trays with a layer of parchment baking paper.

2. Whisk the almond flour with the Swerve, baking powder, and salt in a large mixing container.

3. Mix in the egg, butter, and vanilla extract until incorporated and the dough comes together.

4. Turn the dough out onto a large piece of parchment and pat into a disc.

5. Top it using another piece of parchment. Roll out to ¼-inch thickness. Use a 2-inch round cookie cutter to cut out as many circles as allowed with the dough.

6. Carefully lift the circles using a sharp knife or offset spatula, and transfer them onto the prepared baking sheets. Gather and reroll dough until no more cookie circles can be cut out.

7. Bake the cookies until the cookies are just browning around the edges and firm to touch (for 25 to 35 min.). Remove and let cool completely.

The Peanut Butter Filling

1. In a microwave-safe bowl - microwave to melt the peanut butter and butter using the high setting at 30-second increments, stirring in between, until smooth. Whisk in powder Swerve until smooth.

2. Spread about one to two teaspoons of peanut butter filling onto each cookie's top and place on cookie sheets. Freeze the prepared cookies until firm.

The Coating:

1. Set a heat-proof bowl over a pan of barely simmering water. Add chopped chocolate and butter. Stir until the mixture is melted and smooth.

2. Working with one frozen cookie at a time, add the melted chocolate and toss gently with a fork to coat. Tap the fork firmly against the side of the bowl to remove as much excess chocolate as possible and transfer the cookie to a waxed paper-lined cookie tray.

3. Continue the process with the rest of the cookies.

Note: Try to keep most of them in the freezer as much as possible so that they don't thaw before dipping time.

I said you have one bonus; you have two; here is the keto peanut butter recipe for 17 servings in just 15 minutes!

Homemade Peanut Butter

Ingredients:

- 250 grams or 8.82 oz. of Salted peanuts

- 45 grams or 1.59 oz. Melted butter

Method:

1. Thoroughly blend the fixings, scraping the sides as needed. Blend it until it is creamy.

2. It will remain delicious for two to three weeks - sometimes for even longer times.

Now, you have it all with tons of new copycat ketogenic diet recipes. Enjoy them all without worrying over the carbs; they are all listed!

Lastly, I hope you found the book useful in some way. Please take a moment to post a review on Amazon - it is always appreciated!

CPSIA information can be obtained
at www.ICGtesting.com
Printed in the USA
LVHW041028151220
674216LV00017B/700